Richard Brennan has studied the Alexander Technique since 1983 and has been teaching the technique since 1989; he is the author of six other books on the Alexander Technique, which are translated into nine languages and are on sale world-wide. He has also been featured in many newspapers and magazines including the *Irish Times*, the *Sunday Tribune*, the *Irish Examiner*, *Cosmopolitan*, *Hello*; he has appeared on BBC 1 and RTE 1. Richard is co-founder of The Irish Society of Alexander Technique Teachers (ISATT) as well as being the director of Ireland's only Alexander Teacher Training College, which is approved by the Society of Teachers of the Alexander Technique (STAT). Richard travels extensively throughout Europe and the USA giving talks and presenting courses on the Technique

Other books by Richard Brennan

The Alexander Technique: Natural Poise for Health
The Alexander Technique Manual
Mind and Body Stress Relief with the Alexander Technique
The Alexander Technique Workbook
Stress: The Alternative Solution
Change Your Posture, Change Your Life

BACK IN BALANCE

Use the Alexander Technique to Combat Neck, Shoulder and Back Pain

Richard Brennan

WATKINS PUBLISHING

LONDON

This edition first published in the UK and USA 2013 by
Watkins Publishing Limited, Sixth Floor,

75 Wells Street, London W1T 3QH

A member of Osprey Group

1 3 5 7 9 10 8 6 4 2

Designed and typeset by JCS Publishing Services Ltd

Printed and bound in China by Imago

A CIP record for this book is available from the British Library

ISBN: 978-1-78028-594-8

www.watkinspublishing.co.uk

Distributed in the USA and Canada by Sterling Publishing Co., Inc.
387 Park Avenue South, New York, NY 10016-8810

For information about custom editions, special sales, premium and
corporate purchases, please contact Sterling Special Sales
Department at 800-805-5489 or specialsales@sterlingpub.com

Picture acknowledgements: page 7 Custom Medical Stock Photo/Alamy; 15 Dirima/
Shutterstock; 26 Cultura Creative/Alamy; 31 Henrik Weis/Getty Images; 34 AISPIX by
Image Source/Shutterstock; 48 Yuri Arcurs/Shutterstock; 50 @erics/Shutterstock;
54 MedicalRF.com/Alamy; 63 Image Source/Getty Images; 65 Science Photo Library/
Alamy; 84 Yuri Arcurs/Shutterstock; 93 Tony Hutchings/Getty Images; 100 PhotoAlto
sas/Alamy; 103 Noah Clayton/Getty Images; 108 Superstock/Getty Images.

CONTENTS

Acknowledgements

I wish to thank all the people who have helped in the production of this book: for my agent Susan Mears, who found me a good publisher, for Michael Mann of Watkins Publishing, who has been directly responsible for most of my books getting into print. I would also like to thank the following people who have directly contributed to the content of the book: Dr Nick Mann for writing the foreword; Dr Kieran Tobin and Professor Paul Little for looking over the medical chapter; Sile Chochlain for doing the first and thorough edit; Deborah Hercun at Watkins; Emma Copestake for her help in researching the pictures; and Giora Pinkas, Caroline Martin, Rome Godwin, Veronica O'Shaughnessy, Bill Benham, Sara Shepherd, Katrina Kenny, Stephanie McDonald and Aino Klippel for sharing their stories in the last chapter.

For Caroline

FOREWORD

ALEXANDER TECHNIQUE AND BACK PAIN: A DOCTOR'S EXPERIENCE

Six months before I qualified as a doctor in 1990, while on a medical elective attachment in Sri Lanka, I suffered an injury which changed my life. During my first attempts to learn how to surf I was swept up by an eight-foot wave and dumped, face-first in a diving posture, onto the sea-bed. The facial impact and neck pain were immediately quite severe, but it was only later as I kept spilling drinks into my lap and with persistent numbness in my arm that I realized I had sustained a nerve root injury in my neck. A neurosurgical consultation and X-rays reassured me that I hadn't actually broken my neck and I was able to continue the attachment, but my surfing days were well and truly over.

Over the next twelve years I was beset with constant, increasing, neck, bilateral arm and upper back pain. Following a minor incident the night before my MRCGP exam in 1994, I suffered third-level nerve root pain and weakness in my arm. The subsequent MRI scan showed markedly accelerated degeneration of the vertebrae and discs in my cervical spine, with the expected nerve root compression from bulging discs and osteophytes. The discal bars were also indenting my spinal cord. The neuroradiographer commented, 'You have the spine of a seventy year old.' I was thirty-two!

Although I managed to carry on working as a GP, I continued to suffer unrelenting mechanical and nerve root pain. Around 2000, I consulted four consultant neurosurgeons, who all recommended different operations, ranging from simple removal of a single intervertebral disc, to removal of two or three discs with plating and filler, to replacement of a disc with a prototype 'Cummins' articulating intervertebral joint replacement. My concern about having any such surgery was the increased stresses that would inevitably act on adjacent vertebrae in my neck. I knew that something was still causing large compressive forces to act on my spine even after a decade following the initial injury. Rather than recovering, I was deteriorating. Having found a great neurosurgeon who shared my understanding of the mechanics involved, I was listed for the Cummins joint-replacement operation. It was retrospectively fortunate that, three days before the operation, the pre-op MRI showed that the disc space had completely collapsed, significantly reducing the chances of a successful outcome. After some discussion, we agreed that the best option at that time was to cancel the operation.

I struggled on until, in 2002, there came a point when I became unable to lift my stethoscope to listen to someone's chest. The pain had somehow changed in nature and had become of an unbearable intensity; my right hand had swelled and changed colour, and there were changes to the skin, nail and hair growth when compared with my left hand. I had developed complex regional pain syndrome (formerly – and I think more accurately – known as reflex sympathetic dystrophy). This syndrome is not properly understood in medicine: many doctors still wrongly believe it to be a factitious condition that denotes an excessive individual response to pain perception, mediated solely by the phenomenon of 'central (brain) sensitisation'. I was unable to work for a year after I first developed CRPS. I could not turn my head or look up. I was unable to sit or lie back against any surface; sleeping was a nightmare. The pain from someone hugging me or shaking my hand was excruciating. Eventually, my weak and pain-riddled right arm started to lose its neurological tone and co-ordination and it began to flap limply as I walked.

Since 1990, I had seen a variety of osteopaths and chiropractors, receiving variable treatments, which had afforded differing degrees of transient relief. With increasing desperation, by 2002 I had also tried homeopathy, reflexology, acupuncture and even faith healing. It was ultimately a combination of two brave and iron-handed osteopaths who, by skilfully and forcefully freeing my jammed and displaced upper ribs, began the very slow healing process. In my case, it became apparent that the underlying pathology lay in the mechanical distortion of the sympathetic trunk (a large nerve bundle containing regulatory nerve cells and fibres) as it runs over the upper rib heads next to the spine.

A major impediment to my recovery was that, as a result of the long-standing neuromuscular changes in my spine, minimal movements would cause the ribs and vertebral joints to jam up again, invoking the return of the pain. The spinal neuromusculoskeletal network recalibrates muscle settings over time, such that the dysfunctional settings become registered as 'normal' by the body. My central neuromuscular reflexes and programming had been usurped by years of reacting to, and compensating for, pain and dysfunction that had progressed to encompass my whole spine. I continued to see osteopaths when necessary to unjam my ribs, but I realized that my posture and the way that I was doing things were instrumental in causing the problems to recur.

I first saw an Alexander Technique teacher in early 2002, some time after my wife had attended baby massage sessions at our local GP surgery. My wife had been shown by the visiting Alexander teacher how she was hunching and stooping when pushing the buggy and – in a few easy minutes – was guided into an effortless and more comfortable way to propel the pushchair. The effect on my wife of that one brief intervention was lasting and notable enough for me to want to try the Alexander Technique, although at the time I was more hoping for therapy rather than for tuition. As I have since learned, however, the benefit of being correctly taught the Alexander principles is that they can continue to be employed indefinitely, with continuing benefit.

I found a local Alexander teacher, but I felt that she was not the right person for me and it was then that I contacted Brita Forsstrom, a well-respected member of the Society for Teachers of Alexander Technique in the UK. Within a few sessions, I could sense that beneficial changes were occurring in my body as a result of applying the principles I was learning. I noticed that I could achieve diminution of pain in posture and movement – if only I could hold on to what was happening in the lessons. It took a little longer for me to properly understand and implement the key concepts of conscious inhibition and direction. Brita's gifted hands were an essential component in the initial process of me feeling what was happening in my own body and then developing the awareness and control over how to change it.

One of the effects of neuromuscular recalibration is that we cannot then rely on our own kinaesthetic sense of what is 'normal posture'. Simply put, we all need a mirror to know whether or not our feeling of 'standing up straight' is in fact correct or not. More often than not, it isn't. The Alexander teacher's eyes and hands are therefore essential to provide objectivity in the kinaesthetic reorganization process.

By superimposing Alexander principles over my sub-voluntary postural and pain responses, I gradually became able to undo subtle patterns of gross and postural movements that had been aggravating and helping to maintain the strain patterns in my spine. After an Alexander lesson I would be in much less pain; I felt lighter in my body and consequently my mood. I noticed improved balance, strength and co-ordination and calmness in my movements.

Being bred from the medical model, I tended initially to look for 'tricks' in movements that would help to produce the intended results. As I gained understanding of the concept of 'end-gaining', however, I became less focused on the idea of 'Do it this way, not that way' as the means to an end. It is by consciously inhibiting those very sub-voluntary patterns of movement – by 'not doing' – that I started to become able to 'free up' my body.

It is thanks to a few years of Alexander lessons with a brilliant teacher that I have continued to improve, rather than to further deteriorate, over the last decade since 2002. I continue to have relatively unstable upper ribs, and degenerate and 'sticky' vertebral joints. But importantly, I have no day-to-day pains in my neck, arms or back any more. This is despite a recent MRI scan showing that I still have marked degenerative disc changes, with apparent fourth-level nerve root compression and indentation of the spinal cord itself. If I were to rely on the MRI to assess my status, I would be considered as warranting surgery. However, functionally I am so much improved that I have been able to train, and now practise, as an osteopath alongside my role as a GP.

Osteopathy provides a quick and direct method to 'unlock' the segmental causes of back and neck pain, although the same results may well be achieved in most cases, possibly more slowly, solely by Alexander tuition. The high quality of evidence from the 2008 ATEAM trial (a Medical Research Council-sponsored, large, randomized controlled trial (RCT) of Alexander Technique for chronic back pain) confirmed that the benefits of twenty-four lessons of Alexander Technique significantly outweighed the benefits of normal GP care, exercise and massage therapy, and that – uniquely – *the benefits* (reduced disability and pain scores) *from Alexander Technique were actually significantly greater one year later.* A further rigorous analysis from the ATEAM trial showed that Alexander Technique is also cost-effective. In my perfect world, back pain would be treated in multi-disciplinary medical clinics, with osteopathy and Alexander Technique used side by side to address both the mechanical and dynamic aspects of the causes of back pain. I believe that the huge national and personal burden of back pain could be substantially reduced in this way, even more so by implementing Alexander lessons in school settings, which – by coaching children through the time when much formative change happens regarding posture – could help to prevent the onset of much of the posturally based causes of back pain in adults.

Spinal pain is the single biggest cause of sickness, disability and loss to industry in UK. Physiotherapy exercise treatments have been the mainstay of treatment for chronic back pain for decades, amounting commonly to just brief exercise instruction and advice, but the evidence for benefit from exercise is only mediocre, and those benefits cease as soon as the exercise stops.

It is disappointing that, despite better, more robust evidence for Alexander Technique than for any other modality of treatment for back pain, the government and medical establishment have done little to recognize or to implement the potential benefits of Alexander Technique, for both individual sufferers and for our economy as a whole. The medical establishment continues, completely wrongly in my view, to demedicalize back pain, preferring the paradigm that simple mechanical back pain has no underlying structural or physical cause. While most doctors' reliance on treatments for back pain solely involves advice, analgesia and physiotherapy, I feel that little progress has been made.

Foreword

Alexander Technique can be used both to remedy mechanical spinal pain and to prevent its occurrence/recurrence. Despite the difficulties of rendering practitioner-dependent therapies into RCTs, robust evidence for Alexander Technique now exists academically and empirically. Medicine has yet to recognize this fact, and to overcome the significant institutional biases that exist within the medical establishment. We need to avail ourselves of the most useful tools in order to secure the best outcome for patients and the economy.

I wonder how my life would have been different, had I not hit the seabed head first. Had I known what I know now, had I been using myself in an Alexander way, I may well have hit the ground differently in the first place. For me, it has been a long learning experience. The Alexander principles can be learned in a much shorter time. I have no hesitation in recommending the Alexander Technique and I wholeheartedly welcome this book *Back in Balance* as the first step in eliminating neck and back pain.

Dr Nick Mann MBBS MRCGP MLCOM
Well St Surgery
28 Shore Rd
London E9 7TA
June, 2012

INTRODUCTION

If you are one of the millions of people who are suffering with back pack, I understand only too well what you are going through, because I myself had excruciating back pain and sciatica for many years and was told that I would never ever be able to bend or lift anything, no matter how light, ever again. Standing was painful, as was sitting or walking and even sleeping; in fact, there was no refuge from the pain I was experiencing. I spent a lot of time and a great deal of money on techniques, back aids and treatments that just did not work for me, so I am very familiar with the feelings of frustration and hopelessness that many back sufferers experience. I had the best treatment that the medical world had to offer because my father was a well-known doctor where I lived and many of his friends were consultants and surgeons. I was utterly amazed when at last I found the solution to my long-standing back problem – amazed that the solution was actually so simple. So simple, in fact, that I had completely missed it myself, and so had the dozens of doctors, surgeons and therapists who had been trying to help me over many years. I was so impressed with the power of the Alexander Technique in helping me free myself from back pain that I left my previous job to train as an Alexander Technique teacher. Since 1989, I have been in a very rewarding career helping other people with back and neck pain move towards a life which is pain-free.

The Alexander Technique was the method that was so helpful for me and I hope that by sharing my experience I might reach

1

many other people in pain to tell them that something can be done for them. Unlike other methods the technique does not have side-effects or involve any risk; it is an effective technique which helps you to be more aware during your everyday actions and can help you to reclaim your power to free yourself from back or neck pain. The famous comedian Woody Allen once said: 'More than at any other time in history, mankind faces a crossroads. One path leads to despair and utter hopelessness, the other to total extinction. Let's pray we have the wisdom to choose correctly!' Sometimes having a back problem feels exactly like this – that there is no path that leads to a life free from back pain and many people have given up the hope of ever finding a long-term cure for their back. This book is about a completely different approach from any other method or treatment I have encountered. The basic premise of the Alexander Technique is that the body is very intelligent and knows exactly what is needed to reduce pain. The only trouble is that without realizing it we are constantly putting huge pressures on the nerves, muscles and joints through the way we stand, sit and move, and this pressure prevents healing taking place.

Once you realize how much excessive tension we hold in our muscles, you can then start to release the tension to allow your body to come back into balance. The Alexander Technique is not a quick fix and it does take a little time to learn as it is a re-education of the entire muscular system – a muscular system that is often pulling most of us out of shape. In fact, it pulls our bones and joints together with so much force that it can literally drive the intervertebral discs out of place and onto the nearby nerves. I sometimes say to my pupils that if you did to someone else's back what you are doing to your own you would be arrested for grievous bodily harm! And I mean it.

My only aim in this book is to convey the knowledge that I myself had to learn: a knowledge which freed me from back pain permanently. I can honestly say I have not had a day of back pain in the last 24 years, after having back pain and sciatica every day of my life for over five years continuously. Since teaching the technique, I've also seen many other people from all walks of life become free from back and neck pain by using the ideas and techniques set out in this book. I hope to convey a message of hope to people whose back pain is literally making their life a misery. By the end of the book I hope you will feel renewed hope that at last you will have found a long-term remedy for your back pain. This book is about empowerment: it will point to a means whereby you can heal your own back. It contains many stories from people from all walks of life who suffered with back pain and have been helped by the technique. I suggest you read it from cover to cover and then go back over it slowly a second time to really digest and implement the ideas set down in this book. I sincerely wish you a life free from back pain.

– 1 –

BACK PAIN:
THE MODERN EPIDEMIC

97% of people with back pain could benefit by learning the Alexander Technique – it is only a very small minority of back pain sufferers that require medical intervention such as surgery.

Dr Jack Stern, spinal neurosurgeon and founding partner
of Brain and Spine Surgeons, New York, USA

If you are reading these pages, it is very likely that you have been suffering with back pain either constantly, or intermittently, for a number of years. Well you are not alone, as 80 per cent of the population in developed countries experience back problems at some time. I recently tried to find out how many books about back pain had already been written so I typed 'back pain' into the books section on www.amazon.com and was truly amazed to see that there are over 88,000 books about back pain! That's a very good indication of how prolific back pain has become in our society today. I want to assure you that this is a very different approach: it not just another book about doing 'back' exercises or about improving posture by 'sitting up straight' or 'pulling your shoulders back', nor does it tell you to use lumbar support, a back brace or any gadget that is supposed

5

to alleviate back pain; it is not a book that is trying to tell you that your core muscles are too weak and you need to strengthen them or that there is something fundamentally wrong with your back. In fact, it does not tell you to *do* anything, but rather it will show you than you are probably *doing* far too much with your muscles already without realizing it. If only you could stop *doing* so much you could release the muscular tension, which is so often the root cause of back pain, and your back would get better by itself naturally. This book goes to the core reason as to why nearly half the population in many developed countries suffer with back pain.

According to recent figures,[*] back pain has now reached epidemic proportions, with millions upon millions of people in the UK and USA alone experiencing severe muscular pain every year – most of which is completely unnecessary in my experience, as it is primarily due to poor postural habits while performing everyday actions. In the last decade alone in the UK, the number of people who suffer from back pain has risen from 40 per cent to 49 per cent. In the US, the situation is even worse: in a study published recently[†] it was found that the prevalence of chronic, impairing lower back pain more than doubled in the period from 1992 to 2006. Increases were seen in both men and women of all ages, and across all racial and ethnic groups. In fact, over 4 million people type 'low back pain' into Google every month!

According to the UK's National Back Pain Association, 'BackCare', on average a third of people living in industrialized countries suffer from back pain at any given time, and a staggering 80 per cent of the population of these countries will have disabling back pain at some point in their lives. The Health and Safety Executive in the UK

---

[*]   National Back Pain Association, www.backcare.org.uk
[†]   US Department of Health and Human Services, www.ahrq.gov/research/ju-l09/0709RA14.htm

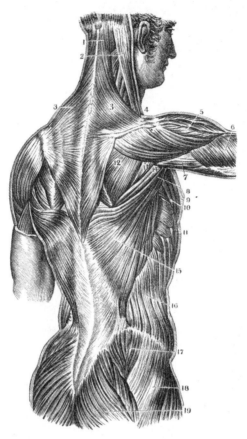

The back is a complex structure and an over tightening of the back muscles can trap nerves or push intervertebral discs out of place.

agrees that back pain is a major problem that will affect as many as four-fifths of people during their lifetime and results in 4.5 million working days lost each year. In the US, the National Center for Health Statistics reports very similar percentages. It says that over 76 million people in the US are suffering from backache at any given moment. The big question is: Why is there such an epidemic of back pain? By the time you have finished this book you will not only know why, but you will also know what steps to take to cure your own back problem and how to prevent occurrences in the future without the aid of exercise or drugs.

It is also amazing that we now have an increasing number of practitioners, perhaps more than ever before, specializing in back problems, most of whom have very good intentions, offering a myriad of solutions for your back pain. This list includes chiropractors, osteopaths, physiotherapists, a wide variety of consultants and back surgeons, yoga teachers, countless pilates and exercise instructors, the use of painkillers, muscle relaxants, anti-inflammatory drugs and a wide variety of orthopaedic aids – yet more and more people are suffering with back pain than ever before, so it is obvious that many of these treatments are not effective *long term*. The simple reason is that most of these treatments try to 'fix' the patient's back without first finding out what the root cause of the back problem is. Please do not get me wrong, I would not like to live in a world without these practitioners and medical remedies, as most of them are offering *short-term* relief for back pain and that is much better than no help at all.

Long-term relief

What I hope to do in this book is to explain why back problems are so widespread today and why many sufferers from back pain are going around in circles without gaining any long-term solution for their back problem. I also hope to offer a practical solution that will alleviate your back pain for good. Anyone with any muscular or skeletal problems other than back pain (such as neck, hip and knee problems) will also find this book helpful, and if you are one of those unfortunate people who have several different aches and pains throughout the body, you will be very pleased to know that one simple solution may cure all.

This book is very different from other books on back pain as there are no actual physical exercises in the book, as many of these, in my experience, often do more harm than good when it comes to back pain. Instead, I would like you to consider the possibility that you may be unintentionally causing the problem yourself. I know that this may sound as absurd to you as it did to me when I had very severe back pain, but, after trying many, many different practitioners and a wide range of remedies, it turned out to be true. I learned that I was the only person who could heal my own back. I did so by using the Alexander Technique, which helped me to become aware of, and change, the postural habits that were directly causing my back problem. If we are actually causing the problem ourselves, it makes perfect sense why most treatments are only effective for a short time. As soon as we have finished the session with the therapist or doctor, most people do not change the postural habits that have caused the back pain in the first place, so it is usually only a matter of weeks or even days before the pain reappears. How can it be otherwise?

Some of the information that you will find here is also included in my other books, for two very important reasons. I am not assuming that you have read my earlier books, so you may have never heard of the Alexander Technique before and therefore need to know the basics of this wonderful technique, and, secondly, sometimes it is only when you read or hear some information several times in different contexts that you really appreciate the actual content of what is being said.

Those suffering with back pain can be put into two categories: those who have been involved in an accident of some kind, and those whose back pain began for no apparent reason. For those in the first category, it may have been a car accident, a sports injury while playing football or rugby, riding a horse or a skiing accident, or it might have started with a fall of some kind. If you happen to be in this category, it may be helpful to ask yourself the following two questions:

- Is it possible that excessive tension was present in the muscles when the incident happened and that it was that tension that caused or contributed to the damage to your back?
- If the body is a natural healing machine, then why is your back not healing?

Although obviously I cannot be absolutely sure, I think that there was probably a good chance that you had excessive tension in the muscles at the time of the accident, perhaps even causing the problem in the first place, and that this same tension may also be preventing healing from taking place. I say 'probably' because so many people are carrying far more tension than is necessary these days.

If your back pain came on for no apparent reason, in my experience, it is again likely to be caused by years of tensing your muscles unconsciously and then one day, for example, you may have bent down to pick up a light object such as a book or newspaper and your back went into a spasm of pain.

Either way, it is the excessive tension in your muscles that is likely to have caused, and is still causing, your back pain and this tension needs to be dealt with if you are ever to be rid of the pain. This may be clearer if I explain how my own back problem and sciatica came about.

My own back problem

I am not only writing from the point of view as someone who has been effectively helping people with back pain for 24 years, but as someone who suffered with an ongoing back problem for many years, so I know what it is like to be in pain over a long period of time. In fact, that is why I came to the Alexander Technique in the first place. My back pain was primarily caused by sitting in a car all day long due to my sedentary profession as a driving instructor. I often spent over 60 hours a week sitting in a car and after several years working at this job, I developed lower back pain. At first, it was an occasional aching back that was relieved by massage or some gentle exercise, but before long I was suffering with such an extremely painful condition that I could hardly walk. The last straw was a minor car accident, which left me unable to work.

My father, who was a medical doctor, was the first person from whom I sought advice, but although he was very concerned about my condition, he could offer me little help apart from painkillers and the standard medical advice of rest. This brought only temporary relief and as time went by even the powerful painkilling drugs I was taking became less and less effective. It was not long before I needed to get back to work, due to financial pressures, but sitting in the car was the worst activity for me as it immediately exacerbated my condition.

I then attended several physiotherapists over a number of years, and although some of the treatments helped for a day or two, my condition got steadily worse and worse. Before long, I was also suffering from sciatic pains that were shooting down my left leg, and I got to a stage where I could not sit, stand or walk without pain shooting through my whole body. It was like a dark wizard in a Harry Potter film administering the 'Cruciatus Curse' over and over again!

Eventually, I saw a series of back specialists, some of the best in the country, who took X-rays and performed various other tests. Although a prolapsed disc was diagnosed as the cause of my problem, no one told me what had caused the disc to be prolapsed in the first place, or how I could get the disc back in place. I was advised that I would have to get used to the fact that I would never be able to live a normal life again and was offered 'pain management'. I did not, however, want to manage my pain – I wanted to be free of it! During the pain management course, I was told that I should avoid bending, lifting and carrying anything at all costs. The pain, however, was still as bad as ever and getting worse. I then saw another surgeon who advised me to undergo surgery to remove the three lowest intervertebral discs, as this, he promised, would reduce the level of pain. Although I initially agreed to this, my father persuaded me to cancel the operation because he was treating people who had undergone similar operations, many of whom were in even more pain than before, and very few were actually any better. So as a last desperate attempt to find some relief from the pain I underwent an intensive course of physiotherapy treatment, even though this had not worked before, and I became an inpatient in a large residential physiotherapy hospital near London. One of the treatments at the hospital involved improving posture and I was told to 'hold myself straight' and 'pull my shoulders back', but this only aggravated my pain instantly – in fact it aggravated the problems of all the other patients in the session too. Although the physiotherapists were obviously doing their best to help, the treatment and exercises they gave me were not helping me at all; in fact, when I was discharged from the hospital, my back pain was worse than ever.

At this stage I started to investigate various forms of alternative medicine. These included the more established therapies such as chiropractic, osteopathy, homeopathy and acupuncture, and then I tried less orthodox treatments such as reflexology, metamorphic technique, aromatherapy, reiki and spiritual healing. In fact, I was so desperate I would have tried practically anything, and while some of these treatments helped to some extent I could only get short-term relief as the severe pain always returned within days of any treatment.

I finally gave up after many years of searching and resigned myself to a life of pain. Up to this point no one, including myself, had considered why the discs had become prolapsed in the first place.

By chance one day I met an Alexander teacher who explained that the Alexander Technique could be very effective in helping back sufferers, like myself, who had tried many other remedies without success. Although I had no idea what it was and was understandably very sceptical after all the other treatments I had received that had failed to help me, I decided to have a couple of sessions to see what it was all about. At this point I was quite desperate as the pain was present day and night and so I felt that I had nothing to lose. I had no idea what 'learning the Alexander Technique' meant. As I had come across the technique in the context of music and acting, being neither a musician nor an actor, I could not really see how it was going to benefit me.

During my first lesson, within minutes my Alexander teacher, Danny Reilly, asked me whether I always sat the way I was now sitting. To be honest, I really didn't understand what he was talking about, so he put a mirror in front of me and I could clearly see that I was twisting to the right, while leaning at least 20 degrees to the left. Yet, despite the fact that I was obviously sitting in a very crooked way, I felt perfectly straight. This was quite a revelation to me. I was amazed that I had never noticed it before and even more amazed that no other person who had tried to help me in the past had noticed it either. Danny set about making a few gentle adjustments to the way I was sitting and two things happened: in my new position I felt completely twisted to the left and leaning way off to the right – yet at the same time my back pain started to ease. He showed me in the mirror how I was now sitting and to my amazement I saw with my own eyes that I was sitting perfectly straight.

After a few lessons the changes in my posture felt less strange and my back pain started to slowly, but surely, subside more and more. It was at this point I realized that when I had been teaching people to drive, I had developed the habit of leaning to the left while twisting my pelvis to the right: this was so that I could see both the road ahead and check to make sure that the learner drivers I was teaching were looking in their mirrors at the same time. Over the years this had become my habit whenever I sat and it was this very habit that had given me all my problems. As the tensions gradually diminished during a series of lessons I also noticed that it was not only my back that was improving: I started to sleep better, my self-esteem and confidence also grew and to my surprise I was gradually becoming happier as well. Within three months I was leading a normal life again and was lifting and bending without any problem at all.

Pain is a warning sign

Many people carry on, as I did, for years with unnecessary pain, not realizing that anything can be done about it. We do, however, need to face up to the fact that we have to take responsibility for our ailments and not expect others to have all the answers. The technique opens up a journey of personal discovery. Pain is simply the body's warning system, which is trying to tell us that something is wrong. By learning the Alexander Technique you will discover what is wrong and how to put it right.

In this book I will show that many back sufferers today are standing, sitting and moving in ways that are putting incredible pressure on their muscles, bones and joints. This muscle tension has often become habitual and unconscious early on in life and as a result most people are completely unaware of the damage they are doing to themselves on a daily basis. From my 24 years' experience as an Alexander Technique teacher, I believe that there is little point in a

People with back pain often lean back even more, which only makes things worse.

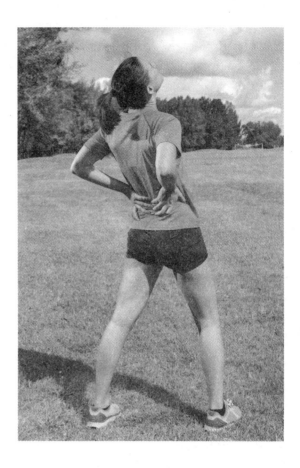

patient having an operation, a chiropractic manipulation or doing a series of physiotherapy exercises if he or she will afterwards continue with the same unhealthy postural habits that caused the back problem in the first place. These postural habits need to be corrected in order to avoid the all-too-common scenario where the back sufferer goes from one therapy to another, searching harder and harder for relief, but without success. We first need to understand that most people's back problem originates from inside themselves.

– 2 –

Understanding the Alexander Technique

Genius, in truth, means little more than perceiving in an unhabitual way.

William James

The story of Frederick Matthias Alexander is a truly remarkable one by any standards. He was always a very practical man – he had no time for theories or for ideas that were not based on practical experience. He did not have a back problem but a voice problem, and understanding how he overcame his difficulty with his voice will be invaluable to you when trying to find the solution to your back problem because the way of finding a solution to each of these different problems is, in essence, exactly the same. Alexander was forced into his search by a problem that was interfering with his profession as an actor and reciter. The problem he had was a recurring and worsening hoarseness in his voice and the solution to this problem led Alexander to discover why so many people have a variety of reoccurring health issues.

The young reciter

Alexander was a successful Australian reciter in the late 1890s with a tremendous determination to become a great Shakespearean actor. He was actually achieving his goal and becoming increasingly successful; as a result, Alexander began to accept more and more engagements, his audiences got bigger, and consequently so did the halls in which he performed. As there were no microphones or any other voice aids in those days, this put more and more strain on his voice, which eventually became hoarser and hoarser. He began to realize that all of his ambitions were under threat because his voice was not standing up to the demands being made upon it.

He approached a variety of people, including doctors and voice trainers, who gave him various medications and exercises, but nothing seemed to make any difference. In fact, the situation deteriorated still further, until on one occasion Alexander could barely finish his recital. He became more and more anxious as he realized that his entire career and all his aspirations were in jeopardy. He grew increasingly desperate and he approached his doctor once again even though previous treatment had not worked. After a fresh examination of Alexander's throat, the doctor was convinced that the vocal cords had merely been over-strained and prescribed complete rest of his voice for two weeks, promising that this would give Alexander a solution to his problem. Determined to try anything, Alexander used his voice as little as possible for the two-week period preceding his next important engagement. He found that the hoarseness in his voice slowly disappeared.

Cause and effect

At the beginning of the performance Alexander was delighted to find that his voice was crystal clear; in fact, it was better than it had been for a long time. His delight soon turned into huge disappointment, however, when half-way through his performance the hoarseness returned, and the condition continued to deteriorate until by the end of the evening he could hardly speak.

The next day, he returned to his doctor to report what had happened. The doctor felt that his recommendation had had some effect and advised him to continue with the treatment. What subsequently transpired proved to be at the very heart of the Alexander Technique.

Alexander refused any further treatment, arguing that after two weeks of following the doctor's instructions implicitly his problem had returned within an hour. He reasoned with the doctor that if his voice was perfect when he started the recital, and yet was in a terrible state by the time he had finished, it must have been something that he was doing to his voice while performing that was causing the problem.

The same reasoning can be made with a back problem: if your back is fine before you do the gardening, drive a car or sit at a computer and it is painful when you have finished a particular activity then it stands to reason that it must be something you are doing during the activity that causes the pain.

This was really a stroke of genius on Alexander's part because, in effect, he stopped relying on other people to give him the answer to his problem and took responsibility for causing his own ailment. As you saw in chapter one I was also causing my own back problem by the habitual way I was sitting in the car, but for many years I had never thought for one second that I was causing it myself. I had been told by professional people – in whom I had put my trust – that there was something wrong with my back: some said that I had a weak or defective back, others thought I had damaged my back somehow, perhaps a fall or even possibly from birth. Not one person gave me any clue why it might be weak, damaged or wrong, and no one told me that I was causing it myself by the way I was standing or sitting. If we can find the root cause for a back problem, which we will explore later on, we can then start to change the detrimental postural habits that keep the back in a painful condition.

So Alexander started to investigate if he might be putting strain on the vocal organs in some way that was unknown to him. Alexander's capacity for original thinking and not accepting anything at its face value was evident even when he was a small boy – he was perceived as a perfect nuisance at the school he attended in Tasmania because he questioned almost everything he was taught. He annoyed his teachers by asking them how they knew that the information they were giving him was correct! There is no way of knowing how many people with back pain have given up looking for a solution for their back problem because they accepted unthinkingly that if medical treatment failed there could be no other solution but to have an operation, which in some cases can do more harm than good.

Using mirrors

In order to observe what he did when he used his voice, Alexander practised speaking in front of a mirror. By observing what he was doing, he soon found that three unusual things took place every time he recited. He observed that he had a tendency to pull his head back, depress his larynx, and suck air in through his mouth. He noticed that at the same time he tended to raise his chest and shorten his whole body. After a great deal of experimentation, Alexander found that if he could prevent the pulling back of his head, the other actions did not occur. This was a major discovery – namely that the interference of the head could so dramatically affect the workings of the rest of his body. This dominance of the head in the hierarchy of the body he later called the 'primary control' and it is the first thing that needs to be dealt with when trying to rectify other ailments in the rest of the body. If you observe anyone with a bad back you will often see that the head is pulled back in many activities that the sufferer performs.

Having discovered what might be causing the voice difficulties, Alexander now started to correct these faults. He simply attempted to do what anyone would do: he tried to do the opposite of what he saw he was doing in the mirror. However, the more he tried to do the right thing, the more frustrated he became, because he found that often trying to do the opposite actually made the problem worse. This is very common when we try to improve our posture: if we think that poor posture is the cause of our back problem, we try to sit up straight and pull our shoulders back, but this only adds more tension to an already tense back.

Alexander soon realized that he couldn't stop these bad habits by simply trying to do the opposite and at last he understood that instead of doing something different, he merely had to stop doing what he was already doing. This is the next vital principle of the Alexander Technique, which goes against all the traditional ideas about correcting back pain. Usually, if something is wrong with our back, we think we must 'do' something to put it right. Instead, with the Alexander Technique, if there is 'something' wrong with your back, you must find out what that 'something' is and decide to stop doing it. This is where the technique differs from all methods of alleviating back pain that I have encountered to date. The common mindset today is that when there is something wrong with your back, a doctor or therapist will undertake the task of trying to 'fix' your back for you without first finding out what is the underlying cause of the problem in the first place. This is a fundamental principle in understanding any attempt to change our postural habits in light of the fact that they are all too often the root cause of the problem. In short, the Alexander Technique will give you the knowledge of how to liberate yourself from the cage of an over-tense muscular system, which may not only cause back pain, but may also contribute significantly to many of the physical, mental and emotional problems that we see in society today. By learning the technique you will rediscover the natural, painless free movement that we all had as children. It is very important to realize that we do not have to learn to have 'correct' posture, but we need to learn how to reduce excessive tension in our muscles so that our beautiful, spontaneous, graceful posture can re-emerge.

Faulty sensory appreciation

Returning to the story of Alexander, he had now reached an impasse. He could actually see what he was doing wrong, yet he knew he couldn't 'do' anything to correct it. By continuing to observe himself he saw that what was happening in the mirror did not correspond at all to what he felt was happening inside himself. Alexander started to see that he could not trust his sense of feeling about where his body was in space or how much muscular tension he was using during any given task. This sense is known as the proprioception or kinaesthetic sense. Up until then, no one questioned the reliability of this sense, a sense that every one of us uses when evaluating how we are moving, where any part of the body is in relation to the other parts or even how much tension there is in our muscles at any given time. Alexander thought that his unreliable sensory mechanism was merely a personal idiosyncrasy and never suspected that anyone else would be having similar problems, but in the first chapter of his book *The Use of the Self* he writes:

> My teaching experience of the past 35 years and my observation of people with whom I have come in contact in other ways have convinced me that this was not an idiosyncrasy, but that most people would have done the same in similar circumstances. I was indeed suffering from a delusion that is practically universal.

Alexander called this phenomenon 'faulty sensory appreciation' and this is the primary cause of our lack of awareness about what we are doing to cause back pain. This makes it crystal clear why other methods that deal with back problems, which do not take faulty sensory appreciation into account, are bound to fail.

Inhibition

Alexander then realized that he had totally underestimated the force of his habits. Like him, we all have very ingrained, stereotyped habits of movement. In my experience it is these habits that are often directly causing our back pain and which we need to examine if any lasting change is going to take place. Alexander had another stroke of genius when he realized that the only place where he could begin to change these wrong habitual patterns was at the moment when the idea came to him to speak or move. Whatever state of tension he was in would get worse from the very moment that he went into action. He clearly saw that the only moment in time where he could change his habits, which were dominating everything he attempted to do, was at the moment that he started to perform the action. This moment in time was the very instant that he was reacting to a stimulus. During everyday activities we react to stimuli with our stereotyped habits, which we have been doing for years. This reaction is done without any awareness or knowledge of what we are doing to ourselves and is an immediate response of the whole self, according to habitual patterns of movement which we have developed from childhood. Because we do what 'feels normal' and right to us we have no choice how we sit, stand or move, and until we learn to choose our movements we can behave in no other way. We are enslaved to these stereotyped patterns of movements or habits just as surely as if we were a pre-programmed machine. Alexander at last realized that he had found the answer to his curious voice problem. He must give himself a moment in order to allow himself a chance of refraining from his usual habit and consciously choose the best conditions when using his voice. He called this 'moment of refraining' from a particular habit or reaction 'inhibition'. The word inhibition as Alexander used it simply means the opposite of volition. It is a moment of withholding consent to automatic reaction. It does not mean suppressing an emotion in the sense in which it is nowadays used in psychoanalysis.

Having effectively prevented the old unconscious patterns of movements from repeating themselves, and having made a break from the reactive, unthinking, mechanical behaviour that was so familiar, Alexander then used his brain for conscious deliberate action by sending mental instructions to the parts of the body which he had been unable to control before. He called these mental instructions 'directions' or 'orders'. He first started to prevent the pulling back of the head that was detrimentally affecting the neck and torso. He gave himself a stimulus, such as speaking, and just refused to respond to it: he gave the conscious messages or directions without actually carrying out a movement. In this way he was preparing new pathways in the brain and eventually he was able to continue the new messages during an actual movement. Over time, the old problematic, familiar patterns were replaced by the new conscious ones, which consequently led to a more co-ordinated, trouble-free working of his body.

Again, in *The Use of the Self*, Alexander writes:

After I had worked on this plan for a considerable time I became free from my tendency to revert to my wrong habitual use in reciting and a marked effect on this upon my functioning convinced me that I was at last on the right track, for once free from my tendency I also became free from the throat and local trouble and from the respiratory and <u>nasal</u> difficulties with which I had been beset from birth.

In the following chapters we will have a look at how Alexander's story can help you with your back or neck problems.

− 3 −

ARE YOU SITTING COMFORTABLY?

People do not decide their futures. They decide their habits and their habits decide their futures.

F. Matthias Alexander

Back pain does not just happen to people – there is a definite cause, a definite reason that we can uncover. In school, most people have learned and can understand Newton's third law of motion, which states that for every *action*, there is an equal and opposite *reaction*. All we really need to do is apply this law to our own back problem. All back sufferers may be very familiar with the 'reaction', which is often debilitating pain, but most have no idea about what 'action' they are doing that causes this. Doctors may tell you that you have a trapped nerve or that a disc is out of place, but they usually cannot tell you *why* the nerve has become trapped or *what* caused the disc to come out in the first place, and this is where the Alexander Technique comes in. It does exactly that – it helps to pinpoint what we are unconsciously doing as we perform our everyday actions that is directly causing the pain. It does not really matter how the back problem originated – perhaps a car accident, a sports injury, pregnancy or simply poor posture – the way we are standing, sitting or moving can exacerbate the pain and prevent an old injury from getting better.

Other theories

There are many theories as to why the vast majority of people living in industrialized society will suffer from back pain at some time in their lives. Some say that back pain is caused by some huge evolutionary mistake. They think that we should still be living on all fours or up in the trees and the very fact we are upright at all is causing all the

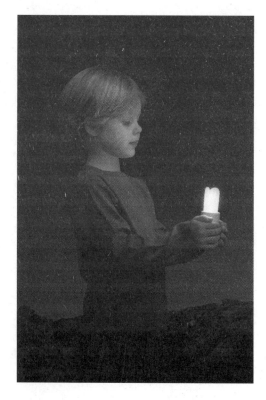

Nearly all of us start out life with a very upright, healthy and aligned spine.

muscular and skeletal problems that we are seeing today. Other people think that back pain is simply a genetic problem that has been handed down from generation to generation. Other people just presume that it comes from a weak spine, which was formed in the womb through some malfunction and has been present since birth.

In my opinion, for the vast majority of people it is none of these at all. The people who believe the fact that we have become upright to be a big evolutionary mistake need to realize that millions of people in underdeveloped countries, who are all walking upright as well, do not experience back pain at all. The proportion of people in vast areas of Africa or India who are suffering from back pain is far less than the number of people suffering with back pain in industrialized countries such as the USA, the UK, Australia and most of Europe. It also very rare for children under the age of five or six to have backache or neck problems and they too are upright. This strongly indicates that it is the way we are living in industrialized society rather than evolution that is at fault.

In response to people who think of back pain as having genetic roots, I say that I have never heard of or seen evidence of a back-pain gene. On many occasions, however, I have seen children copying their parents. If one or both parents have poor postural habits, it is highly likely that their children will copy those habits. The hunched shoulders and arched backs that many adults have from postural habits are acquired by the children themselves, who will surely pass them on to the next generation. So while research may quite rightly come to the conclusion that back pain runs in families, as far as I am concerned it is not because of genetics, but due directly to imitation.

People who think that weak backs are embryonically formed are simply underestimating the power of nature. There may be the odd occurrence of a spine not forming properly during fetal development, but a figure as high as 80 per cent of the population is highly implausible.

The sitting habit

I encourage you to read the following pages with an open mind because a major reason why so many of us get back pain seems so blindingly obvious that it gets overlooked time and time again. I want you to forget all the reasons you have been told in the past that may be the cause of your back pain. I personally found with my own back – as well as the many people that I have taught as an Alexander teacher – that posture and the way we perform actions is the fundamental cause of back problems for most people. The very first important question to ask is why so many adults have detrimental postural habits, such as rounded shoulders or an overarched back, when nearly all children under the age of five or six have perfect posture? The answer can be found in our sitting habits. In most industrialized cultures we like to sit down. Many of us spend as much as 75 per cent of our waking lives sitting on chairs: we sit to eat, we sit at the computer, we sit in the car, the bus or train when travelling to work, and we sit in our homes when relaxing. In fact, according to the *Daily Telegraph*,* the average person in the UK spends more than 14 hours a day sitting down – since we sleep for an average of eight hours per night, British people are therefore only on their feet for less than two hours a day. It emerged from the study that the typical working adult spends 4 hours and 17 minutes at their desk and, once home, they will sit down again to use a laptop or home computer for another 2 hours and 25 minutes, and a further 2 hours and 27 minutes parked in front of the TV. These figures don't include

---

* 'Britons spend more than 14 hours a day sitting down', 19 May 2012.

the time sitting while travelling to work. I cannot imagine that it is any better in the USA where 'drive-in' movies, banks, churches, takeaways and supermarkets have become the norm. The less we stand and walk, the less we feel like standing and walking: it becomes a vicious circle. It is not only the fact that we sit so much, it is also the fact that we rarely give a thought to what we sit on – yet what we sit on will surely affect the way we sit. In my experience most of the chairs we are sitting on are not synchronized with how our body is designed and this is a major factor in causing poor posture, subsequently leading to back pain. It is interesting to realize that back pain and neck problems have reached epidemic proportions in all countries where sitting has become the norm. Chairs and desks are the most common ergonomic factors that have encouraged poor posture, so let's have a look at the way most of us sit.

School chairs

Many people do not realize that the chairs they sit on can actually shape the form of the human body so severely that some people are bordering on deformity. Driving for long distances or spending long hours at our computer, on badly designed car seats and office chairs, can practically cripple us, so that by the end of the journey or a day's work we can barely straighten up afterwards, yet we rarely blame the chair – we blame our back! It is fairly obvious that the designers of most kinds of chairs have not studied the way that the body is designed to work. Some chairs are not only uncomfortable, but can actually be harmful when used for long periods. Some years ago I was invited to Middlesex University in the UK to talk about the Alexander Technique to students in their final year of a degree course in furniture design. Before I began my lecture, I asked the students what they considered to be the most important aspect when designing a chair. Nearly all of them gave me the same answer: 'Colour!' I was a little surprised because I had expected them to come up with something more technical, such as the height of the chair or how the chair supported the human frame. I was intrigued by their answer and wanted to know more. 'Why colour?' I asked them. 'It's obvious,' they said, 'if you designed the best chair in the world, but covered it with lime-green material nobody would buy it.' And then I realized that most furniture designers are putting a great deal of emphasis on whether the chair *looks* aesthetically pleasing, but are paying little attention to the design of the human body. A chair may have inviting curves and may even initially feel comfortable for short periods, but the same chair often offers inadequate support and actively encourages poor posture in the long term and may directly cause unnecessary strains and stresses to the spine. But why do we put up with or even buy this kind of chair in the first place?

To answer that question we have to go back to our school years, when we all had to sit on uncomfortable school chairs – we did not have a choice. Imagine telling a teacher that the school chair you were sitting on was uncomfortable and you would like a replacement. It does not take much imagination to know what the answer would have been. To understand why the standard school chair is the root cause of so much future back problem, we need to look at the whole scenario.

During our years at school, most children will sit for over 15,000 hours, which is a huge amount of time, especially if the chair design is putting unnecessary strain on the muscles and joints. It is simply not natural to sit for prolonged periods, no matter how good the chair is, because our body is designed for movement, not for keeping still.

The main reason why the typical school chair is bad for children's posture, and ultimately their backs, is the fact that the back of the chair

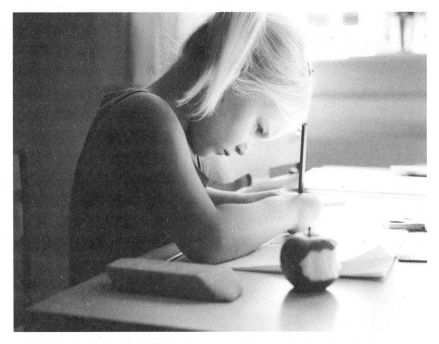

Hunching over school desks for long periods can often lead to back pain in later life.

slopes backwards and the horizontal part of the chair, which takes most of the weight of the body, is also sloping backwards. So the key parts of the chair are oriented backwards, yet we expect the child to move forwards in order to be closer to their school desk to read and write – this makes no sense whatsoever. I am not sure whether to call the standard design of school chairs ridiculous or just absurd! The bones that we sit on are often referred to as the sitting bones or sit bones (the medical term is *ischial tuberosities*); they are the lowest part of the pelvis. If you look at the image of the pelvis on page 54 you will notice that these are rounded and you do not need a degree in physics to realize obviously that if you put this rounded surface of the sitting bone on the backward-sloping base of a chair, gravity will cause it to rock backwards, causing pressure on the lumbar area. (If you place a marble or golf ball on a typical backward-sloping chair or car seat you will see immediately what I mean.) This backward and downward force that is exerted on the pelvis puts enormous pressure on the lumbar area of the spine, which is exactly the area where many people feel the pain in their backs. These types of chairs actually prevent children from bending in the hip joint, which they need to do in order to lean forward while reading and writing at a desk. Once they find that they are unable to rock forward on the sitting bones because it is very difficult to rock 'uphill', or they cannot bend at the hip joint because the whole pelvis is collapsed, they will have to find another way to reach the desk – and this usually involves actually bending their whole spine which starts to put pressure on the discs all the way up the spine. This bent back eventually becomes a permanent habit in everything schoolchildren do, as can be seen in so many teenagers when they sit, stand and walk – they start to have a bent back even when there is no need. The reason why nearly all school chairs are designed in this way is because it allows them to be stacked without the danger of falling over; while that may be more convenient for the cleaners, it is a disaster for the children's natural upright posture. In fact, because of the amount of damage that these chairs are doing to millions of children's back I often refer to them as 'weapons of mass destruction'.

When children sit on this kind of low, backward-sloping furniture, which is the norm in every school I have ever been in, they usually have no option except to tense up many of their muscles in order to just maintain an upright posture. It is not hard to see that this excessive tension and the habit of bending of the spine are the seeds of future back problems, and in my mind is a major contributing factor for the huge number of people who are suffering with back pain that we see in our society today.

The children themselves do everything they can to counter the influence of this backward-sloping chair – let's just follow what happens to the child when they go to school at the age of four or five and are forced to sit in a chair. No child likes to sit down for very long, and many immediately find the chair itself very uncomfortable; for reasons already explained, it is not suited to their natural posture so the first thing nearly all children try to do is get up and move around. Ask any primary school teacher who looks after five year olds – he (or she) spends a great deal of time making sure that the children stay in their chairs. Children have a natural ingenuity and intelligence when it comes to posture and body awareness, and so their next instinctive strategy is to try to counteract the 'falling backwards' movement produced by the chair by tilting themselves forwards, raising the back legs of the chair off the floor as they do this. This is an intelligent strategy as it corrects the backward slope of the chair seat, making it level or slightly forward-sloping, and this helps them to maintain an aligned, upright posture with much less effort. Nearly all children do this, but instead of being curious as to why so many children are tilting their chairs forwards, we just tell them exactly what we were told ourselves: 'Don't swing on the chairs – you will break them!' The damage to the child's posture is not even considered or noticed. The children still do not give up: they then often develop other techniques to counter the effects of the backward slope, such as sitting on a foot, which also has the effect of raising the pelvis. This is just another way of enabling them to pivot on the sitting bones, again keeping an aligned and healthy spine; however, it is often actively discouraged in case the blood flow to the leg is restricted.

Over and over again the child is prevented from doing what comes naturally to them and eventually the child gives up, and they learn to endure sitting in backward-sloping chairs for literally thousands and thousands of hours while at school. Sooner or later, most if not all of them slowly but surely begin to slump as their back muscles become more and more fatigued. In effect, what we are doing is this: first we ruin children's posture by making them sit on badly designed furniture, and then, in our ignorance, we chastise the children for slumping. It is pure madness! As their posture begins to deteriorate over the years, many children are told to 'sit up straight' and 'put your shoulders back'; the only way to do this, however, is to overarch the lumbar spine and contract many of the powerful back muscles that are already tense. Worse still, the children then begin to think that this is the way they ought to sit. Unfortunately, this rigid posture becomes fixed within the body and can often remain with them for the rest of

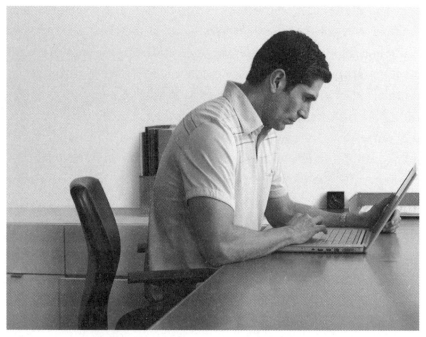

After 10 years of sitting hunched over school desks the bend in the upper back becomes the habit in everything we do. And this habit is present in many of our activities.

their days, causing their muscles and joints to become progressively stiffer or more painful as time goes on. According to figures quoted by Sean McDougall, who is the chair of the charity Pain UK, as well as a former trustee and CEO of BackCare, 21 per cent of children experience back pain by the age of 16, and 15 per cent of all children under 16 seek medical attention to deal with the pain.

This has been backed up in a report by the National Back Pain Association in October 2005, which states: 'Sustained poor posture, which is probably the key environmental cause of back pain in children and adolescents, results from a combination of factors, the most significant of these seems to be the inappropriate furniture at school.'

Very few people are aware that backward-sloping furniture causes as much damage as it does; in fact, currently there is a proposed European standard for chairs and tables used in educational institutions (prEN 1729-1), which has increased the specification for the sloping base for school chairs to increase from -5 degrees to -10 degrees. This can only compound the problem if it is implemented.

Car seats

Unfortunately, the problem of these backward-sloping chairs is not confined to schools as the general design is practically universal. Just take a look at your car seat and you will probably find that the base as well as the back slopes backwards. You may remember that my problem was caused primarily by the car seat I was sitting on. Not only was I leaning to the left while rotating to the right but I was also sitting on a backward-sloping car seat for nine or ten hours a day. After I had trained to be an Alexander teacher I wrote to all the major car manufacturers, such as BMW, Mercedes, Audi, Ford, Toyota, Mitsubishi, VW, etc. I explained about my back problem being partly caused by the design of their car seats. Only VW replied, and all they said that they were happy with the design of their car seats. While the car manufacturers may be happy, a lot of people climbing out of their cars after a long journey are anything but happy, often in a lot of pain and hardly able to stand up straight.

These days even children's pushchairs and car seats are also following this trend of sloping backwards. Just look around you: the base of nearly every car seat, office chair and sofa slopes backwards and nowadays some even have the added problem of a firm 'lumbar support' pushing into your lower back at the same time. In fact, we have all become so used to these backward tilting chairs that they now feel normal and it is what we have come to expect – it is hardly surprising that many people have acute back pain after a long drive or after sitting in these kinds of chairs for a long time. It really is a catalogue of disasters, but fortunately for us the solution to this problem is a simple one.

Improved sitting

To solve this problem all you need to do is to alter the base of the chair so that it is no longer sloping backwards. This can easily be achieved by using a wedge shaped cushion. You can test this out for yourself at home by placing two books, about 5 centimetres (2 inches) thick (old telephone directories are ideal), and placing one under each of the back legs of the chair. This should make the base of the chair flat or, better still, sloping slightly forwards, and will encourage you to pivot on your sitting bones when leaning forwards. Obviously, the books are not practical for everyday use, but wedge cushions can be obtained in many outlets. Make sure that the wedge you buy is made from good-quality hard foam. Those made from softer foam may be cheaper, but they are much less effective. Many back sufferers that I have come across have got immediate relief from using a wedge cushion or a forward-sloping chair. If you get a wedge cushion, it is important to sit on it for only one hour on the first day and then gradually build up the amount of time you spend sitting on it. This allows time for your postural muscles to get used to a new and improved way of sitting. After about 3 to 4 weeks you will be able to sit on the cushion comfortably for as long as you like.

Even better still, buy a chair which you can adjust the angle of the base so that you can have it in different positions to suit the different tasks you are doing. Details of websites where you can get good-quality wedges and adjustable chairs can be found on the resources page in the back of this book. It is important to note that the wedges and forward-sloping chairs are only to be used while you are sitting involved in an activity and not particularly when you are sitting to relax. The times when it most helpful to use the wedge cushion are when you need to lean forwards: for example, when writing, working at a computer, eating your meal or while driving.

Another important factor when considering the design of chairs is height. A very interesting statistic is that today children are now on average four inches taller than their 1950s counterparts, yet furniture is now typically eight inches lower. It is often also the case that the height of a chair is virtually the same for all chairs, yet human beings are very different in size. So it is also very important that your chair is the correct height for you; a rough rule of thumb is that your chair needs to be a third of your height. It is important to realize that, although changing your chair is a very good start, it will not necessarily alter the postural habits you have become accustomed to that have been caused by the chair itself. To change the postural habits that have been caused by the backward-sloping chairs, you will need some Alexander lessons as well.

– 4 –

Improving Posture

As any action or posture long continued will distort and disfigure the limbs; so the mind likewise is crippled and contracted by perpetual application to the same set of ideas.

Samuel Johnson

After changing your chair to a more supportive seat, you will need to start to undo the postural habits that have probably been acquired over many years. Before trying to improve our posture, however, it is very important to understand what exactly we are trying to improve and how to go about it in a constructive way. Today many people think of improving posture as merely adjusting a shape or position by increasing the tension in the muscles. In fact, Alexander did not like the word posture as he found it too limiting and too static: he wanted a term that was more dynamic, which included movement and even our emotional state as well as the way we think. The term he preferred was 'the use of the self'. So when I use the word posture in this book please understand I am also talking about something much more profound than just a static position or shape – for me posture includes the way you are presenting yourself to the world physically, mentally and emotionally. Plato once said: 'The cure of the part should not be attempted without treatment of the whole', so it is not just a matter of one or other part of body being out of place – we also need to think of posture as being all-inclusive and is a direct result of how we think, move and feel. They are so unified that by changing one of these, you change them all.

Improving posture

You may have been trying to improve posture already without success; this might be because many people go about it in a way that just makes the situation worse. If you merely try to sit up straight by pulling your shoulders back, you will probably just be overarching your back and this will almost certainly make your back pain worse than ever. We are actually living in a muscular 'suit' and by tightening one set of muscles, you will be affecting the whole muscular system. Changing posture is actually a process of 'unlearning' or 'undoing' and there is no way that you can 'do' an 'undoing'. To effectively improve our posture we simply have to eliminate the habits we are doing that cause our poor posture in the first place. We need to understand that excessive tension is the main cause of poor posture and anything we 'do' will increase that tension and only make the situation worse. We do not even have to work out what the right posture is, all we have to do is to find out where we are holding tension that is causing poor posture and then let that tension go – then the 'right' posture or movement will just happen by itself. Young children naturally have good posture, but they are not *doing* anything to get that graceful posture nor are they going about their daily actions working out what the best posture is. They do not hold a position or shape for very long either, they are always very dynamic. Good posture is simply a part of them and it is a part of us too, if only we can all stop interfering with what is natural.

So let's have a look for the moment at how many of us have improved posture in the past and then find a new, more effective way. As we saw in the last chapter, most of us have come out of school having spent many years sitting on badly designed chairs that have encouraged us to hunch over a school desk – not surprisingly our posture has taken a turn for the worst. We may look in the mirror one day and see that our shoulders are pulled forward and our spine is rounded at the top. What most of us do as a reaction to this is what we have always been taught to do: we pull our shoulders back to straighten our spine. We do this with muscular tension. The reason that our shoulders are pulled forward and our spine is rounded, however, is because the muscles at the front – namely the pectoralis major and abdominal muscles – have become shortened over a long period of time and this has being caused by the habitual contraction of the muscles concerned. In our efforts to correct things, we try to pull our shoulders back and to stand up straight. We do this by tensing the back muscles, namely the trapezius and the erector spinae. We never think for one second about the tension in the front muscles that was causing the problem in the first place, and consequently we only add more tension in our back muscles. In effect, all we have done when trying to improve our posture is to engage in a tug of war between the front and back muscles – a war that no muscle can win, in which both sets of muscles are held in a constant state of tension. This common scenario can be seen frequently in people with back pain. When we have a look at young children with good posture, however, you can see they are holding very little tension in their bodies. In fact, it is the lack of tension that allows for the free and graceful movements that we call 'good posture'. So in order to improve posture we simply need to release the tension in the front muscles that is pulling us down in front, and then there will automatically be less tension in the back muscles.

This is not as easy as it sounds, because we have become so accustomed over many years to holding this tension in the muscles and often we cannot even feel this tension ourselves. This is another vital point for those with back pain because, despite the fact that excessive muscular tension in the back muscles is often the root cause of back pain, this tension has become so habitual that it goes unnoticed by the person in pain. This is partly due to the fact that the kinaesthetic and proprioception sense, which informs us of the amount of tension in our muscles, receives its information partly through the muscle-spindles in the muscles themselves. These muscle-spindles are very small mechanisms whose function is to convey information about the state of the muscles from the muscles to the brain, and then the brain sends information back to the muscles as to what they should do. However, if there is excessive tension present in the muscles, these lines of communication between brain and muscle are, in effect, put out of action, and we can no longer feel what we are doing. This explains why, despite our back being in pain, we cannot feel the tense muscles that are causing the pain. This tension often goes unnoticed by the medical profession for the simple reason that muscular tension does not show up on either X-rays or MRI scans.

Understanding posture

When looking at how to improve our posture, it can be very helpful to understand some of the basic principles as to how our muscular system works. Within the muscular system, there are two very different types of muscle that are responsible for doing two very different jobs. There are muscles that organize our posture and those that organize movement. While it is true that any muscle can at times do either task, some muscles are more suited to the task of performing movement while others are better at the task of maintaining posture.

The primary task of the first type of muscle is to keep us upright against the ever-present force of gravity, and they are often referred to as 'postural' muscles. We rarely have to think about maintaining our balance as we go about our daily activities – it is all done for us by an amazing system of intricate postural reflexes, without any conscious effort on our part. We can stand for a long time without these muscles tiring because they are 'fatigue resistant'. They are automatically triggered by powerful reflexes throughout the body, which produce the appropriate muscle tone for any given task. As soon as the stimulus for these reflexes is removed, these muscles automatically relax. We are often not aware of this process as it often takes place subconsciously.

By contrast, the 'phasic' muscles are more suited to performing activities and they work in a very different way to the postural muscles. If you want to raise an arm or a leg, you must first make a conscious decision to move the limb and then determine how much you want to lift it. The muscles you use in this way react quickly, but also tire quickly. You can try this for yourself by holding your arm out to your side horizontally: within a few minutes you will be able to feel the muscles in your arm begin to tire. These differences become clearer when you look at the chart below which compares the different types of muscle and their function:

Postural Muscles	Phasic Muscles
The primary function of these muscles is to support and keep us upright against the force of gravity	The primary function of these muscles is to perform movements

Postural Muscles	Phasic Muscles
They have a predominance of muscle fibres that are reddish in colour	They have a predominance of muscle fibres that are whitish in colour
These red fibres contract relatively slowly and are referred to as slow twitch	These white fibres contract quickly and are referred to as fast twitch
These muscles are fatigue resistant and therefore take a very long time to tire	These muscles are not fatigue resistant and therefore often tire quickly
These muscles are activated by our postural reflexes and therefore do not need the conscious mind to activate them.	These muscles are always activated by the conscious mind

The crucial point here is that most people try to improve posture by *deliberately* tensing the phasic muscles as they 'sit up straight' or as they 'pull their shoulders back'. This strategy will never work because they are simply the wrong muscles for the job and as a result they will tire very quickly and we will not be able to maintain even what we think is a 'good position' for very long. So, even with the best of intentions, if we use the phasic muscles to improve our posture we will fail every time and we will soon find ourselves with even worse postural problems than when we started, as we will have even more muscular tension than ever. Even if someone had plenty of willpower and was prepared to put up with the discomfort, over time these muscles would become fatigued and increasingly immobile, eventually causing more pain than ever.

The key to good posture is to learn to reduce the amount of tension in the over-worked phasic muscles so that the postural muscles can start to do the work that they were designed for. This is exactly what

Alexander meant when he said that if you stop doing the wrong thing, the right thing will happen by itself.

Alexander lessons

What takes place during an Alexander lesson may vary depending on your own requirements and the way your teacher puts across the information. If the teacher has not been personally recommended to you, it is worth having one lesson from two or three different teachers to see which way of teaching suits you best. Various organizations will supply a list of qualified teachers and details can be found in the resource section at the end of the book.

Your first lesson may be slightly longer than subsequent lessons as details of how and when your back pain started will need to be discussed. You may also be asked if you have other health problems apart from back pain. It would be helpful to mention any accident or trauma that you feel may have contributed to your back pain. Some teachers also take some time to discuss the principles and history behind the technique. After this, the teacher usually observes how you are sitting, standing or moving to see what postural habits you may have that are contributing to the pain you are experiencing. Then, while sitting, standing or lying, your teacher may use their hands to gently move a limb or head and ask you not to help, while he (or she) assesses your muscles for excessive tension. When muscle tension due to an inappropriate postural habit is discovered, your teacher will ask you to think about releasing tension while performing a particular action, and consequently you can begin to become aware of the habitual tension that you may never have noticed before. In this way, the phasic muscles become less tense and the postural muscles start to be used for the job for which they were intended.

It is difficult to describe some of the experiences that people have had during or after their lessons. For me it was a wonderful feeling of lightness and ease and I felt that all parts of my body began to work in unison with each other. It can give people a sense of peace and oneness and many people describe the feeling as 'walking on air', or as 'having all the joints well oiled': it is simply the feeling of letting your body work as nature intended without the presence of back or neck tension. Most importantly of all, many people feel a substantial reduction in back pain. Following your first lesson, this feeling may only last for a short time, but with subsequent lessons this will last for longer and longer periods. I will talk more about this experience in chapter thirteen.

When you have learned how to let go of the muscle tension that has often accumulated throughout your body over a number of years, you will begin to relearn various movements that will help to prevent the tension from returning. You will relearn different ways of walking, standing, sitting and bending that put far less strain on your body. If you are an office worker, a musician, a sportsperson or have an occupation that is causing specific problems, your teacher will help you to analyse those activities so that you can learn to do them in a different and pain-free way. After a course of lessons, you will be much more aware of all of your actions and will often clearly see what was causing your back pain so that you can avoid any future occurrences.

– 5 –

THE POWER OF HABIT

Change involves carrying out an activity against the habit of life.

F. Matthias Alexander

We all have personal postural habits when sitting, standing and moving. Not all habits are bad; in fact, we need many of them to function efficiently in life. We do not want to have to consciously think about every movement we make, as we need our conscious brain to be taking on other tasks, and so we utilize the unconscious part of our brains to do the work for us. Learning to drive a car is a good example: most learner drivers cannot understand how an experienced driver can simultaneously steer, indicate, change gears, brake and accelerate and look in the mirror *and* talk to a passenger and wave at their friends! If we take the example of first learning to change gears, we all had to use the conscious part of our brain: we had to *think* about taking our foot off the accelerator, then *think* about putting the clutch down, *think* about which gear we were in and *work out* where the gear you wanted was and perform the movement, bring the clutch up to biting point and then *think* about putting your foot back on the accelerator. Using the conscious part of the brain takes so long that often the car has stopped by the time this action has been completed.

So by repeating the movements over and over again we learn to do them more quickly – in other words we get into a habit of changing gear, and experienced drivers can change gears in a second or two and hardly have to think consciously about what they are doing. The whole process has become automatic and therefore habitual. Just look at professional musicians and notice how quickly their fingers move as they play their instruments; most of this is totally automatic – they could not possibly consciously think about every movement they make. In the same way, many of the actions we make are habitual, and whereas many of them may do no harm, some of them do, and these are the ones that need changing as they can often cause back problems. It is useful to think of developing habits as being like making a path through a jungle. The first time you walk the path it is very difficult and may take quite a while for you to cut the growth; the second time is still difficult but less so. The more times you walk the path the easier and quicker it will be. To get a sense of how strong a habit can be you might like to try this following exercise.

Just fold your arms in your usual way so one hand is tucked in under the opposite arm and the other hand is resting on the opposite upper arm.

Now just reverse the way your arms are. Most people find this very strange or uncomfortable and some find it impossible to do.

Bending our backs

In the same way we have habits that feel totally normal, yet they are directly causing us pain. Without realizing it we often use our spine in a way that it was not designed for. A good example of this is the very common habit of bending our spines instead of our ankle, knee and hip joints – many people with back pain do this thousands of times before they even notice stiffness, tension or pain, which is why we do not immediately connect the way that we are moving with the pain we are experiencing. In the same way, the clutch in a car will only wear out after riding it over and over again and not the first time you do it. Many of us are bending our spine rather than using the actual joints of the body that were specifically designed for bending. It is ludicrous and makes no sense at all, but that is what most of us do. This way of bending our backs may happen hundreds of times a day and we have no idea that we are even doing it: this is because

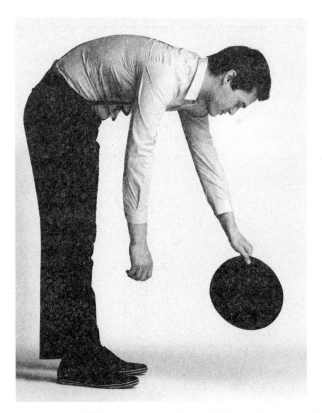

In contrast to young children many adults bend from the top of the hips instead of the joint. This can lead to chronic back pain.

it has become a habit over the years and just feels right and totally normal to us. In fact, this way of bending is so common in society we become oblivious to these habits even in other people and they just look and feel completely normal to us, but if you compare the way small children bend to most adults you can see a very clear difference.

In fact, the movement of bending the hip joints has become so unnatural for many people that when asked to point to their hip joints, a large percentage will not know or point to an incorrect place such as the waist area at the top of their pelvis. Bending in the wrong place now and again will usually not present much of a problem, but bending our spines over and over again until a strong habit is formed is a gross misuse of this incredible structure and is only asking for trouble.

Sitting up straight is unhealthy

Another common unhealthy habit is the one we have already mentioned: the habit of standing or sitting up straight while we pull our shoulders backwards. It is a habit that we were often taught to do to counter the habit of slumping after bending over school desks for many years (due to the badly designed school furniture). Because we were probably taught this by a parent or teacher, we have just presumed that they know better than us and therefore it is the right thing to do. However, this way of sitting or standing causes our muscles to be very tense and gives us the idea that we should have a lumbar curve in our spine at all times, which is really not the case. Again, just look at children and indigenous people while they sit or squat: their backs are very straight and there is no hint of a curve in the lumbar area. The spine is a movable structure and has many shapes, one of which is very straight. If we keep that lumbar curve in

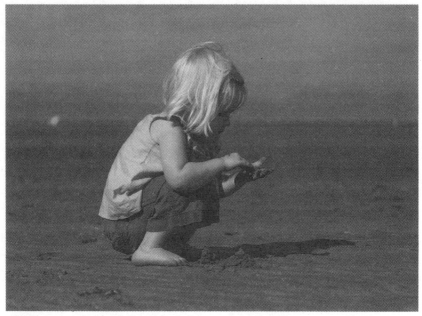

Children naturally bend at the hip, knee and ankle joints.

our spines all of the time, we are setting ourselves up for a life of back pain. Many car seats and other chairs have a lumbar support and people with back pain are often given a lumbar roll by a therapist, which, in my experience, can often exacerbate a back problem.

Most of us do not even realize we are using our body in an unhealthy way even when we are riddled with pain. The simple reason is that any habitual movement, even one that badly harms the body, eventually starts to feel right to us. In Charles Duhigg's book *The Power of Habit* there was an interesting case of a product developed by Procter and Gamble that would eliminate nasty smells. They had spent a vast amount of money perfecting their product, which worked very well, even eliminating the smell of a skunk, but people were not buying the product and they just did not know why until they approached a woman who owned nine cats. The researchers visited the woman's home in Phoenix, Arizona and could all smell the stench of the cats as they were approaching the front door. When the scientists walked inside the house the smell was so overpowering that one of them was very nearly sick. The woman who owned the nine cats, however, was so familiar with the overpowering odour that she was rarely aware of the smell herself any more. She had become so used to it that that her brain no longer consciously registered the odour. You may have had a similar experience yourself when visiting a friend's house where there is a strong cooking or wood burning smell; the smell is very obvious to you the moment you step in the door, but not to your friend.

In the same way, we have become anaesthetized to many of our postural habits too. Many people with back pain are sitting, standing and moving in ways that are causing damage to their back muscles, discs and joints, but have no idea that they are doing these movements. It is much easier to see other people's habits than our own. We sit, stand and move in a way that is familiar to us, irrespective of whether it is harmful. Next time you are out and about just take a good look at the way that people are moving. They may be throwing their hips forward, leaning backwards, hunching their shoulders and throwing their heads backwards onto their spines, usually without any awareness of what they are doing to themselves. It is very useful to compare the movements of adults compared with young children; you will usually see a vast difference. As we saw, Alexander had exactly the same problem with his voice: even though he could see in the mirror that he was pulling his head back; because of the strength of the habit it took a great deal of practice of consciously deciding not to do this habit before he could successfully recite without doing it. Alexander was very opposed to doing repetitive exercises as a way of helping alleviate pain as he realized that when we do these exercises we are often still doing them with all our habitual tendencies and this only makes a habit stronger and harder to get rid of.

Changing habits

To change a habit that is harmful we must of course be aware that we are doing the habit in the first place and that alone can be difficult enough as our habits feel so right and normal to us. The best way of finding out what these habits are is to have Alexander lessons, as this is the quickest and most direct method. The Alexander teacher will help you to discover the personal habits that you have developed over many years and will help you to identify the ones that are directly causing your back or neck pain. It is not a case of replacing your habits with another set of habits: it is more a case of learning to let go of the habits and then consciously choosing more efficient and less harmful ways of moving. We can also observe ourselves in the mirror as Alexander did, and we now have other technological aids, such as iPads, video cameras and mobile phones, which can record our habitual movements. While using this technology can be a good place to start, many people get a surprise when they see their movements recorded, because the way we feel we are moving can often differ a lot from the actual way we are moving. Another useful way of becoming more aware is to observe other people's habits and ask yourself: 'I wonder if I do that?' Changing a habit is not as easy as it sounds as we feel drawn to perform actions in our old way and, like the metaphor of cutting the path though the jungle, not only do we now have to cut a new path, but we also have to refrain from going down the old path. There are so many examples of how to change a harmful habitual movement that it would be impossible to list them all in this book. But let's take a moment to look at some of the most common ones.

Picking up an object

Earlier, we mentioned how many people bend their spines instead of their hip, knee and ankle joints, so let's start by looking at this habit. If you have a video camera or iPad you might like to use it for this exercise. To become aware of how you bend to pick up an object you can do the following awareness exercise:

1. Place a book, a pen or your mobile phone on the coffee table or chair.
2. Walk away from it for a few metres and then go and pick it up in your usual way without thinking too much about it. Do not try to do it in the 'correct' or 'right' way as you need to catch your unconscious habit.
3. As your hand touches the object, just stop completely and ask yourself: 'Exactly what am I bending? Am I bending more in my knees, hips and ankle joints, or am I bending my back or neck?' If you're still not sure, you might use a mirror, video camera or ask a friend or relative to observe you and give you feedback.

This simple procedure will give you some idea of whether you are putting your back under strain every time you bend. We not only bend to pick things up, we also bend when sitting down. If you look at the illustration on page 54, you can see that the hip joint is quite different from where the top of their hips are located, even though many people will point to the top of the hips instead of where the hip joint really is. In fact, if you look carefully at the illustration you will see that the top of the hips is directly in line with the disc between the vertebrae lumbar 4 and lumber 5, which is the very disc that gives many people problems. By bending at the top of the pelvis we are in reality bending our spines rather than the hip joint and will consequently put a lot of pressure on the lower discs and sacroiliac joints. To locate your own hip joints, just place a finger in the groin area and then bend your knees and ankles; you should feel the hip joints moving. Now try bending the knees in such a way that they move away from one another. You might find that this feels quite strange at first, but that is a good sign because any unhabitual ways of moving will often feel unusual if we all have become accustomed to certain stereotyped ways of moving. I have found that allowing the knees and hip joints to bend instead of the spine can dramatically reduce the incidence of back pain. The only advantage of bending the

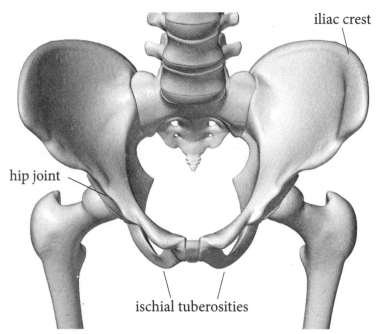

You can see here that the hip joint is quite different from where the top of their hips are located, even though many people will point to the top of the hips instead of where the hip joint really is.

back instead of the knees that I can think of is that it is slightly quicker and it is often the busyness of life that has caused many detrimental habits to occur in the first place.

Sitting up straight

As we saw in chapter four, sitting up straight is a common habit that causes a lot of back pain. Again, the best way to find out how much tension sitting up straight causes is to actually do it. As you are reading these words pull your shoulders back and sit up straight and you should feel the lumbar curve become exaggerated. Can you feel your muscles in the shoulders and lower back over-tightening. A great many people who come to me with back pain are doing exactly this and when they are able to stop doing it the back pain often subsides immediately. When people stop pulling their shoulders back and arching their back, they often feel very slumped down in front when in actual fact they are much straighter than they feel. We learn to do this habit as a consequence of the constant shortening in the front muscles, initially caused by hunching over our books at school and college. In my experience this shortening in the front muscles is often the primary cause of back pain, because we have to use the back muscles to counter the muscles that are pulling us down in the front. I even tell people who come to me with backache that they don't have a back problem – they have a front problem!

During an Alexander lesson, your teacher will help you learn how to release the muscles in the front as this can be very tricky to do by yourself without an increase of tension. A great many gym exercises actually try to strengthen the front muscles such as the pectoral and abdomen muscles and these are the very ones that actually pull us down in front. This strengthening only shortens the front muscles even more, causing the habit of pulling down in the front to become even stronger and subsequently makes the back muscles work even harder, causing even more pain. I found with both myself and many of my pupils that one of the most effective remedies for the habit of pulling down in the front and feeling that we should be sitting up straight is the semi-supine, which will be covered in chapter nine, as this helps to release tension in both the back and front muscles and eventually you won't feel the need to sit up straight any more.

Standing up straight

Standing up straight is a very similar habit and again can put an enormous strain on the back muscles, and often this habit will cause the back to start hurting within a few minutes. You can see this for yourself if you stand side on (at 90 degrees) to a long mirror and then stand up straight. When you look in the mirror, you may well see that you're not straight at all, in fact you may be leaning backwards as much as 20 degrees. This action of leaning backwards increases the tension in the back muscles, which in turn can put huge pressures on the discs and joints of the spine. I don't think that anyone would disagree that leaning backwards for a back sufferer is only asking for trouble, but I have found that so many people with back pain are doing just this without any awareness at all of what they are doing.

Leaning back while walking

In fact, not only do we lean back when sitting or standing, it seems we also lean backwards as we are walking. At a recent conference, there was an interesting presentation by Alexander teacher Bob

Britton. He first showed some film footage of people walking around San Francisco just before the 1906 earthquake and then he showed some footage of people walking down the same street 100 years later. It was evident that the people walking at the beginning of the twentieth century were walking much straighter than those a century later, as the more recent footage clearly showed that most people were now leaning backwards while walking. These actions of leaning backwards while sitting, standing and walking are very common habits in our society today, yet, according to Alexander, we are all able to throw these habits of a lifetime away in a few minutes if we just use our brains.

So how come we have all these postural habits without realizing it? Surely our body should give us some warning that we are harming ourselves? Well the answer is: it does! Pain is the warning that we are doing something harmful to ourselves. However, we do not interpret back pain as a warning to us that we should change our postural habits: we interpret it as 'I have something wrong with my back and I need someone to fix it for me.' A good analogy of this was reported in a newspaper some years ago. An American woman arrived at Heathrow Airport in London from New York. She rented a car as she wanted to visit relatives in Scotland and proceeded up the M1 motorway; however, the car was not driving well as the engine was very noisy and had no power, and could do little more than 30mph (48km/h). When the woman got to Edinburgh she took the car back to the car rental company and complained bitterly that there was something very wrong with the car. She reported that it had taken her at least twice as long as expected to get to Scotland. A mechanic checked the car and could find nothing wrong with it. The woman would not accept the car back and tried to show the mechanic what was wrong. At that point, it became evident that she had never driven a car with gears – she had always driven a car with an automatic gearbox. So she had put the car into first gear and drove the car with her foot right down on the accelerator for over 400 miles (640 km) and didn't realize for a moment that she needed to change gears! Of course the car was very noisy and didn't go very fast – any car would have behaved the same! So, there was no problem with the car – the fact was that the driver was not driving the car as it had been designed to be driven. In *exactly the same way* we do not 'drive' our bodies in the way that they were designed; most of us completely 'misuse' them for many years before our back and neck pain arises. The spine is a rotary structure and so turning the spine left and right is usually no problem at all; it is only when we bend the spine that the problems start, because it is not designed to be used in this way. We need to simply rediscover how the body is intended to be used – any four year old will show you how if you observe them moving around.

– 6 –

FAULTY SENSORY AWARENESS

The right thing to do would be the last thing we should do, left to ourselves, because it would be the last thing we should think it would be the right thing to do. Everyone wants to be right, but no one stops to consider if their idea of right is right. When people are wrong, the thing that is right is bound to be wrong to them.

F. Matthias Alexander

One of the main, but little-known, reasons that our habits go undetected for so long is because of what Alexander called 'faulty sensory appreciation'. If we are ever to change the habits that are the root cause of our back pain, it is imperative that we take this into account when we are trying to rediscover our natural movement, which can put us on the road to recovery from a back problem. As we saw in the last chapter, pain is merely a sign that something is wrong and we need to find out what that 'wrong' thing is. We all presume that if we 'feel' that we are sitting or standing straight then we are straight. We trust our feelings to tell us where we are in space and how much muscle tension is in our body at any given time. However, Alexander discovered that the exact opposite is true for many people: most of us perform the majority of our actions with a faulty awareness of what we are actually doing. Although we may be absolutely sure we have a particular posture or are moving in a particular way at any given time, the reality is that we may well be doing something entirely different from what we think. It is really no wonder that back pain is so rife in our society. It is not until we catch our reflection in a mirror or shop window that we realize how different we are physically from the way we feel we are. It was only because Alexander was using mirrors to get to the root of his voice problem that he realized that what he 'felt' he was doing and what he was actually doing were two very different things.

At first Alexander thought that he was suffering from a delusion that was his own personal idiosyncrasy, but the more he helped others the more he realized that he was suffering from a delusion that was practically universal. In fact, Alexander used to tell his new pupils: 'Don't come to me unless when I tell you you're wrong, you make up your mind to smile and be pleased.' He also said that the correct thing to do to improve the way we use ourselves is often the very last thing we would ever think of doing, because the instrument through which many of us are experiencing the world (i.e. our body, mind and emotions) is faulty, so it is continually giving us inaccurate information. Most of the usual advice for back pain is to perform a set of exercises or take a specific drug, or use a certain type of back aid. The truth is that we need to stop *doing* something to alleviate the pain, not just do something on top of what we are already doing. If a man with a headache was constantly banging his head against a wall, would we advise some pain killers, a crash helmet, or tell him to go bang his head against a softer wall? Of course not – we would naturally tell him to stop banging his head on the wall and that would certainly improve and probably even cure his headache. Like that man, most people do not have a bad back; we are just doing something bad to it. If you can recognize what that bad thing is, you could be well on the way to solving your back problem for good.

Another good example of this is a driver who has a habit of constantly pressing down on the clutch when driving and as a result keeps wearing out clutches. Does he need a car mechanic or a driving instructor? The answer is a driving instructor, because he obviously needs to be taught to stop the habit of riding the clutch and then his problem will go away. In the same way, most people with back pain usually do not need a doctor or therapist or medication, they just need to be taught a different way of standing, sitting or moving that does not harm their backs. In fact, Dr Jack Stern, spinal neurosurgeon and founding partner of Brain and Spine Surgeons of New York publicly stated that he thought that 97 per cent of people with back pain could benefit by learning the Alexander Technique and that it is only a very small minority of back-pain sufferers that require medical intervention, such as surgery – and he is the surgeon!

The sixth sense

As well as having the five senses of sight, hearing, smell, taste and touch, we have an internal sense as well, which for the most part goes unmentioned. This internal or interoceptive sense gives us information about balance, posture and co-ordination, and is the result of several body systems working together. In order to achieve balance and good co-ordination we require information from this internal sense to determine where our body is in space and how we are moving. This information is received and organized by the brain. If the information – or our interpretation of this information – is faulty, which it so often is, then we will constantly be adopting certain positions and movements because they 'feel right', even though we are so often doing something entirely different to what we think we are doing.

It is the interoceptive senses of kinaesthesia and proprioception that Alexander was referring to when he invented the term 'faulty sensory appreciation', but why, when and how did they become faulty? The answer is perhaps because many of us now have far more stimuli to cope with than our ancestors, which can cause our muscles to be in a state of continual tension. If we are receiving too much information our brain suppresses or screens out much of the information from the inner senses to prevent itself from becoming overloaded. If our muscles are constantly in a state of tension, it is also likely that these internal senses cannot efficiently receive the necessary information as the muscle receptors themselves are not be able to work effectively. So the brain itself will not be receiving some of the information that is needed for efficient posture and movement.

As a result, the interoceptive senses can become unreliable and start to give us faulty information about where we are in space. When we stand, sit and move in unbalanced and unco-ordinated ways we build up even more tension in the muscles. As this tension becomes more and more ingrained over the years, we can become totally unaware of how or what we are doing. In other words, we get caught in a vicious cycle: being unable to feel our own muscle tension because our feedback senses are not working properly – and our feedback senses not working properly because our muscles are too tense. Another related issue is that our sense of balance can also be affected. In the inner ear there are semicircular canals that are the organs responsible for balance and equilibrium. The semicircular canals consist of three ducts arranged on three perpendicular planes. These semicircular canals are filled with fluid called the endolymph and when we move our bodies this fluid moves as well. Its movement is detected by hair-like projections called cilia, and then this information is sent to the auditory nerve, where it is processed by the brain. If we are constantly pulling our head back and downwards onto the spine, as many people do, the information that gets sent to the brain about our orientation will be adversely affected. It is not unusual for a person to feel their head is off-balance or crooked once it has been put perfectly straight during an Alexander lesson. This feeling is simply because the fluid in the semi-circular canals changes to a different level. Alexander training can also affect the level of the eyes and during the first few lessons some people may feel as though they are looking slightly upwards compared to their usual gaze.

Without realizing it, many of us take our poor postural habits and faulty sensory awareness into every action we perform, with catastrophic consequences. Even worse, we often bring those habits and faulty sensory appreciation into our practice of various forms of

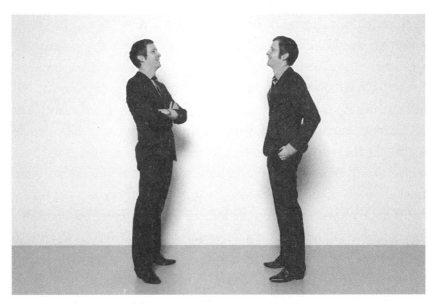

As is the case with the man on the left, many people do not realize that they are leaning backwards, which puts a huge strain on their spine.

physical exercise such as yoga, pilates, physiotherapy exercises, gym work, running and various sports that are supposed to do our back some good when, in actual fact, they often make matters worse than ever. Over the last 24 years, I have talked to a great many doctors, physiotherapists, fitness and sports instructors, yoga and pilates teachers, manual handling trainers and ergonomic instructors, yet not one of them was even aware of the existence of faulty sensory appreciation. I am totally convinced that this is the main reason why the conventional treatments for back pain rarely have any lasting effect. So, no matter how good the therapist is, if we return to the same detrimental habits after a treatment we cannot really expect any long-term improvement.

In all my 24 years of seeing people with a wide range of back problems, I have never come across a person who was not suffering from a faulty sensory awareness and not one of these people even knew that faulty sensory awareness existed. In all good faith, we may be carrying out a series of instructions given to us by the doctor or physiotherapist, but because of our unreliable kinaesthetic sense we will often be performing them totally incorrectly. As we saw, even the simple instruction to sit up straight is often done by overarching the back, which ends up anything but straight. Another good example of this is in the manual handling instruction when lifting. Many people are taught that the way to lift is to 'bend the knees and keep the back straight', and it's easy to misinterpret this instruction to mean 'keep the back vertical' or 'keep the back rigid'. So many people are trying to lift heavy objects while trying to keep their backs vertical and this action alone is enough to cause serious harm. Just look at young children: every time they bend to pick something up, they always bend their knees, hips and ankle joints and although their back stays beautifully straight, it is not vertical – in fact quite often it is 45 degrees forward from vertical.

Many of us don't give any thought to how we move: we simply move in the way that feels normal, comfortable and right to us, no matter how much strain it puts on our back.

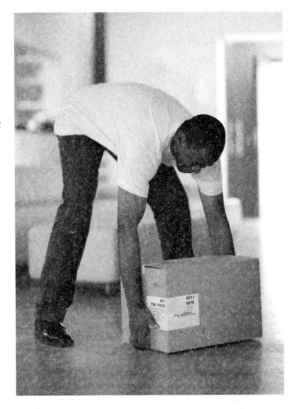

The only reliable way of finding out what we are actually doing is to seek verification from an outside source, such as an Alexander teacher, mirror or video camera. It is only by getting reliable feedback that we can have a chance to first see and then relinquish our harmful habits. For all we know we may be doing all sorts of contortions, but be absolutely convinced that we are perfectly straight. Another example of this can be found at any hair salon: when the hairdresser tells their clients to put their head straight the client often puts their head onto one side and the hairdressers then has to come and manually straighten the head for them, after which many people feel like their head is lopsided.

Awareness exercises

You can try the following observation exercises at home in order to gain a practical understanding of the meaning of faulty sensory appreciation:

Exercise one
1. While looking straight ahead, and *without looking at your feet*, place your feet exactly 30cm (12in) apart.
2. Still without looking at them, place your feet parallel to each other, if they are not already this way. In other words both feet should be pointing straight ahead.
3. Now look at your feet to check if their actual position matches your inner sense of their position. Next you can look at your feet as you place them parallel with one another and 30cm (12in) apart. Do they feel as straight as they look?

Exercise two
1. Stand with your eyes closed and place your arms and hands pointing straight ahead and parallel with each other.
2. Turn your index fingers inwards so that they are pointing to each other.
3. Keep your eyes closed and move the fingers towards each other.
4. See if you are able to touch the two fingers together without looking.

Exercise three
1. Once again close your eyes.
2. Place your arms and hands straight out in front of you so that they are horizontal and then turn the palms of your hands inwards so that they are facing each other.

3. Now see if you can bring your hands together so that all the fingers and the thumbs meet symmetrically and the tips of fingers are touching their counterpart.

You can also start to become aware of yourself while you are sitting and standing. As you are reading these words, notice which parts of you are making contact with the ground or chair. If you are standing, note whether there is more pressure on your heels or your toes, or whether there is more pressure on the outside or inside of your feet. If you are sitting, note whether there is more pressure on the left side or the right side of the pelvis, and if your feet are on the ground supporting you, or do you have them tucked under the chair? Notice where your head is –is it balanced on top of your spine or do you tend to let it drop as you are reading these pages? By becoming more conscious of where the weight of your body is, this can give you vital clues about where your body is in space and how much tension you are holding in your muscles.

Many of us don't give any thought to how we stand, sit or move: we simply move in the way that feels normal, comfortable and right to us. The first thing we need to do is to improve our awareness of everyday actions so that we can find out exactly which muscles are over-tensing as we go about our daily activities. The key to improving balance, co-ordination and movement, and consequently alleviating your back pain, is to become more conscious of what you are actually doing and thinking while you perform your everyday actions. Many of us have had incorrect training when it comes to posture and that training needs to be unlearned. Perhaps this quotation from Socrates, 'All I know is that I know nothing', would be a very good place to start when learning the Alexander Technique.

– 7 –

PAUSING BEFORE ACTION

What lies in our power to do, lies in our power not to do.

Aristotle

By now you may have started to become aware of some of your habits that have directly caused excessive tension and pain, and if so it is obvious that you will need to refrain from continuing these harmful habits and choose different ways of moving if ever you are to escape from back pain for good. 'Inhibition' is the key to doing this and is perhaps the most important of all the principles of the Alexander Technique, for without it there can be no change. Marjorie Barstow, one of the very first teachers that Alexander trained, said: 'Inhibition is the activity by which the old habit cannot take place.' As we saw in chapter two, inhibition was the term that Alexander used to refer to the moment of stopping so that he could withhold consent to the automatic reaction that was causing his voice problem. Inhibition is simply the opposite of volition. The word 'inhibition' has been commonly used to describe a self-imposed suppression of behaviour or emotions ever since Sigmund Freud used the term in his writings on psychoanalysis, but this is not how Alexander meant the word to be used. When using inhibition in an Alexandrian way there should be no suppression at all as we are just creating a space in which we can think and make a reasoned choice as to which is the most favourable action at any given moment in time. The 2012 *Oxford English Dictionary Online* describes the word inhibition as 'a restraint on the direct expression of an instinct' or 'the slowing or prevention of a process or reaction'. The act of inhibiting before performing an action for someone with back pain is simply an opportunity to prevent the habit that may be the direct or indirect cause of their pain, as well as giving them a chance to perform a different movement that does not aggravate their condition. A common example that we have already mentioned is the action of bending the spine instead of the hip joints. Although most people would agree that this is not a good way to bend, as it puts a great deal of pressure on the intervertebral discs, we still need a moment of inhibition to prevent the old unwanted habit occurring automatically and instead consciously choose to allow the hips, knees and ankle joints to bend instead of the spine, allowing a more natural and less harmful way of moving. It is important to point out that the new way of bending is not just making the joints of the legs to bend, but also allowing a release of tension, and is done by means of what Alexander called 'directions', which will be discussed in the next chapter.

In his book *Man's Search for Meaning*, the Austrian neurologist, psychiatrist and Holocaust survivor, Dr Victor Frankl, wrote a very good description of what Alexander meant by the word inhibition:

Between stimulus and response, there is a space.
In that space lies our freedom and power to choose our response.
In our response lies our growth and our happiness.

In that brief moment between a stimulus and how we respond lies the power to turn our life around for the better, and this is exactly what a moment of inhibition can offer us. If we can give ourselves that moment between a stimulus and our reaction, to really choose how we respond to different situations as we go about all our daily actions, rather than be moving in a habitual way with no conscious thought whatsoever, we can really give ourselves a chance to move in a new way that will help us get out of pain. There are many proverbs and sayings that encourage us to do just this, here are a few examples:

- Look before you leap
- Think on the end before you begin
- Fools rush in where angels fear to tread
- Second thoughts are best
- More haste less speed
- Failing to plan is planning to fail
- Prevention is better than cure
- Good and quickly seldom meet

I am sure that you will agree that these sayings are sound advice, but so few of us actually apply them when it comes to the way that we co-ordinate and balance ourselves as we move around on this planet. The following exercise can demonstrate the difference between an ingrained habit and a conscious movement:

Awareness exercise

1. Observe an object that is lying on the ground and without thinking walk over and pick it up.
2. Now repeat the action, but this time just stop for a moment and consciously work out what is the best way of performing that action without hurting your back.

3. Did you notice a difference and if so what was it?

You can repeat this exercise when getting up out of a chair, eating your food, walking or any of the dozens of your everyday actions.

Although our brains can be used as instruments for action, they can also be used as instruments for inaction. The ability to delay or inhibit our responses until we are adequately prepared is the only way of relinquishing our poor postural habits and starting to rediscover easy, natural ways of performing different actions. It is important that the moment of pausing before acting has nothing to do with freezing or performing actions slowly.

Instinctive inhibition

One of the best examples of natural and instinctive inhibition is the behaviour of a cat. You can observe this even in a domestic cat, when it first sees a mouse. It does not immediately rush and capture its prey, but it waits until the appropriate moment in order to achieve the highest chance of success. It is interesting to realize that while cats are fine examples of inhibition, balance and control, they are at the same time one of the fastest creatures on earth. The cat's ability to pause is instinctual; in other words, it is an automatic function of the subconscious brain. Man also has this potential, but in our case it needs to be performed through conscious choice, and it is this difference which defines a clear line between man and the animal world. Life has become so busy for many of us that pausing for a moment is now, more than ever before, necessary in order to delay our instantaneous reactions to the many stimuli that bombard us each day, and to enable us to cope better with our rapidly changing environment.

Conscious inhibition

If we are ever to change the habitual movements that are the root cause of back pain, we have to make a conscious decision to refuse to act in our old automatic and unconscious patterns; that is, to say 'no' to our ingrained habits of use.

By inhibiting our initial instinctive action, we start to have the choice to make an entirely different decision and therefore we can begin to move in a different way. This may be harder than it seems, because although the way we move may be the cause of our pain, our habits often feel normal and 'right' to us. Even pausing for a moment may feel alien to us if we have the habit of rushing all our movements, but inhibition is an essential and integral step when practising the technique. Alexander summarized it thus:

> Boiled down it all comes to inhibiting a particular reaction to a given stimulus – but no one will see it that way. They will see it as getting in and out of a chair the right way. It is nothing of the kind. It is that a pupil decides what he will, or will not, consent to do.

If you are able to prevent yourself from performing your habitual actions, then you are half-way to your goal of having a pain-free life. To refrain from an action is as much an act as actually performing an activity, because in both cases the nervous system is used. It is also possible, and indeed desirable, to inhibit any unwanted habits and tendencies, not only before an action takes place, but also during any given activity. The following exercises will help you to see what it feels like when you do not react immediately to a certain stimulus.

Exercises

1. Every time the telephone or the doorbell rings, pause for the amount of time it takes to take two breaths before answering. Although this is a very simple exercise it is very hard to do for many because most of us have been taught to move immediately without thinking.

2. Whenever you find yourself in a heated discussion or an argument, try counting backwards from ten to one before responding. This is a useful exercise in inhibition and it will give you time to think about what you really want to convey.

3. Choose a simple activity, such as cleaning your teeth, cutting a loaf of bread or loading the dishwasher, and occasionally stop completely for a moment or two and be aware of any excess tension you may be holding in your body.

In this way inhibition can also help you to become more aware of habitual movements.

Slipped disc

One of the most harmful tendencies that Alexander observed in himself was that he was constantly over-tightening his neck muscles, which pulled his head backwards and down onto his spine. Initially, he presumed that this phenomenon was merely a personal idiosyncrasy, but later observations showed him that this was not the case at all – this tensing up of the neck muscles was very commonplace. This habit of pulling back the head on to the spine invariably leads to a compression of the intervertebral discs in the neck or lower back, or both, and causes a shortening of our entire structure.

This downward pressure on the spine may well be one of the major reasons for a variety of back problems, as it can squeeze a disc out of position and this in turn can lead to a disc pressing on a nerve. The spine is made up of many bones called vertebrae. These are roughly circular and between each vertebra is a disc, made of strong rubber-like tissue, which allows the spine to be fairly flexible. A disc has a stronger fibrous outer part, and a softer jelly-like middle part called the nucleus pulposus. The spinal cord contains the nerves, which transmit messages from the brain to and from various parts of the body, and is protected by the spine. Nerves from the spinal cord come out between the vertebrae and the discs. For a prolapsed disc (commonly called a slipped disc), the disc does not actually slip out of place, but rather the nucleus pulposus is pressurized out through a weakness in the outer part of the disc. A prolapsed disc is also sometimes called a herniated disc. The bulging disc may press on nearby structures, such as a nerve coming from the spinal cord, and inflammation can develop around the prolapsed part of the disc. Any disc in the spine can prolapse; however, most prolapsed discs occur in the lumbar part of the spine (lower back). The size of the prolapse can vary, but as a rule, the more the disc is out of place, the more painful your back is likely to be.

Many doctors, physiotherapists and even back specialists are unaware how common this habit of contracting the neck muscles is. The pulling back of the head onto the spine nearly every time we move can often be, in my experience, one of the main causes of back problems. The head is quite heavy (approximately 12lb or 5.5kg) and frequent jerking backwards onto the spine can obviously have a very harmful effect on the neck, back and rest of the body.

This action of pulling the head back is another very good example of what Alexander called 'misuse' and because most people are unaware that they are doing it, or that this habit is causing their back problem, they will understandably continue with this habit, which in turn prevents the back from healing. It is like having a cut and rubbing that cut hundreds of times a day: it is obvious that the cut will never get better. That is exactly the reason that many remedies that offer a solution to a painful back will only last a short time. How could it be otherwise if we continue to perform the same habit that caused the problem in the first place? There is nothing wrong with many other treatments or therapies for back pain – the only problem is that without changing your postural habits as well, you are in effect just throwing your money away. The pulling of the head backwards also significantly interferes with our general co-ordination and balance, which can be so severely affected that we will be forced to hold ourselves in a rigid fashion to stop ourselves from falling over. In other words, when we come to move, we can actually be working some of our muscles directly against other muscles, causing our whole muscular system to be full of excessive tension. It is not unlike continually driving a car around with the handbrake on.

Awareness exercise

To demonstrate that the head is pulled back by excessive tension of the neck muscles during a movement, follow these steps:

1. Sit in a chair.
2. Place your left hand on the left side of the neck, and the right hand on the right side of the neck, so that the two middle fingers are just touching each other at the back of the neck (at the base of the skull).
3. Stand up in your usual way.
4. Then sit down again in your usual way.
5. By being aware of the pressure on your fingers, while you are sitting down or standing up, you will be able to detect any

pulling back of the head. Watch for a feeling that the head is being pressed back into the hands. This indicates neck tension and the head being pulled back.

6. Perform the exercise several times as you may well notice more tension on the second or third repetition.

If we are able to inhibit this unconscious habit of tensing up our neck muscles, then we will put our whole body under far less stress, especially our back muscles, and this may well help discs to go back into place and reduce any inflammation that may be there.

Awareness exercise

Another exercise you might like to try is to stand with both arms resting by your sides. Take a moment to be aware of what they feel like. Do they feel the same or perhaps does one arm feel longer, heavier, freer than the other?

1. Without thinking, lift your left arm up to the side so that it is level with your shoulder. Hold it there for a moment or two and then let the arm drop back slowly to the side. Now repeat the same action again with the right arm, but this time first inhibit your action for a few seconds and become more aware as you are raising the arm up. After a few seconds lower the arm down, again with awareness.
2. Notice if there is any difference between arms after you have performed this exercise; people often experience a feeling of lightness or that the second arm is a different length.
3. Repeat the same exercise, but this time reverse the process, pausing before raising the left arm.

Inhibition is the natural antidote to the increasing stress that we are having to deal with in our daily lives. We are expected to achieve more and work faster in a speed-orientated environment. We are no longer encouraged to do things in our own time anymore and are often rushing to fit in with someone else's schedule. Back pain can often be caused by a person being under too much pressure: I often ask a person who comes to see me whether they were in a hurry when the pain started and 99 per cent say that they were rushing for one reason or another. When rushing around, all of our muscles are in a state of tension and any actions performed in these circumstances may well be asking for trouble.

A man once came to me in a lot of pain; he had damaged his back while bending in a hurry. He was suffering from a prolapsed disc and was in severe pain, which was so bad that he had to spend three months lying on the floor before he came to see me. During that time, he could hardly move without experiencing excruciating pain. He was the sort of person that always did things in a quick manner: he always took a shortcut, as it could take seconds off the journey or the job. When lying on the floor and gazing up at the ceiling for three months, he realized that he now had to pay back all those seconds he had saved. For anyone who has a habit of rushing, the moment of inhibition can be priceless. Jacob Bronowski in his famous book on evolution, *The Ascent of Man*, talked about inhibition as a crucial ability for the whole human race and went so far as to say that our entire existence in the future depended on it:

We are nature's unique experiment to make the rational intelligence prove sounder than the reflex. Success or failure of this experiment depends on the basic human ability to impose a delay between the stimulus and the response.

– 8 –

DIRECTIONS

The Alexander Technique is the discovery by F. Matthias Alexander of the natural rhythm within the human body which exists in the sensory and motivating nerve circuits. This essential rhythm has become distorted in most people and such distortion becomes the principal cause of most of the ill health and distress of many so-called mental and physical diseases.

Patrick Macdonald

The second vital part of practising the Alexander Technique is to be able to give yourselves what Alexander termed as 'directions'. These directions are definite orders or instructions that you consciously think of, and your brain relays these messages to your body. Like inhibition, using directions has the effect of preventing the very action that may be putting unnecessary pressure on your joints, nerves or discs. In the quotation above, Patrick Macdonald, one of the very first Alexander teachers that Alexander himself trained, talks of the distortion of a natural rhythm of the body. This distortion can be detected by an Alexander teacher throughout the body, often as a muscular contraction – a pulling down or a pulling in of the entire body. In extreme cases, they can also be visually detected as a slumped or contracted posture. The directions help to restore this natural rhythm, which has a much more expansive, unrestrained and spacious quality. For this reason, you will find that most of the Alexander directions include the words 'lengthening', 'widening' or 'expanding', which help to prevent the very common contraction caused by over-tense muscles. During Alexander's years of experimentation, he realized that he had never once given any thought to how he directed himself during an activity and, like him, many of us simply move in a habitual way that feels 'natural' and 'right'. Now, by inhibiting for a moment, we can have a chance to prevent these unconscious stereotyped patterns from repeating themselves. Having made a space between stimulus and our response, we can now use these mental instructions to gain conscious control of parts of ourselves that previously have been working habitually.

On page 20 in his book *The Use of the Self*, Alexander described 'giving directions' as: 'A process which involves projecting messages from the brain to the body's mechanisms and conducting the energy necessary for the use of these mechanisms.' It is possible to use directions in two ways. Firstly, you can direct *specific* parts of yourself: for example, you can think of your fingers lengthening. Secondly, you can direct your *whole* self, such as when thinking of your entire structure lengthening. Alexander often instructed his pupils to 'come to their full stature' when giving a lesson. You can also direct yourself as you are moving through space by consciously deciding where you are going and how you intend to get there. It is important to realize that giving these directions is an actual experience and you will need some Alexander lessons to learn how to give them to yourself. I personally have found it is very difficult to give these directions without the experience of specific quality of muscle tone that a trained teacher can impart, simply because, when first learning how to give directions, nearly everyone tries too hard and actually 'does' something rather than just imagining or thinking. When this happens, a person increases the tension even more without realizing it. When we think of the Eiffel Tower or Stonehenge we do not have to 'do' anything with our muscles in the process; we need to think in exactly the same way when giving directions. Don't forget Alexander took many years to work all this out and we can save ourselves a lot of time and trouble by going to a teacher when we are learning the technique.

The primary control

As we saw in chapter two, Alexander discovered that the way his head moved affected the rest of his body – he realized that this phenomenon was caused by a primary control of the working of all the mechanisms. This primary control mainly involves the muscles of the head, neck and back, and these need to be in a free relationship with one another for this primary control to act effectively and without hindrance. The overall purpose of the primary control is to act as the main organizer of the body and to govern the working of all of our muscles and mechanisms; it makes the control of our complex human organism comparatively simple. It is the dynamic relationship between our head and the rest of our body, and Alexander teachers often refer to it as 'the head–neck–back relationship'. It is important to point out that this relationship is not one of position, but one of freedom of the head in relation to the rest of the body.

When, due to excessive muscular tension, the head is pulled back and down, the primary control is interfered with and as a consequence all our actions become harder to do. This in turn can interfere with other muscles and reflexes throughout the body, which can result in a lack of co-ordination and balance. A good example of this can be seen in horse-riding. If a rider pulls the horse's head back with the reins the horse loses balance and co-ordination and its movement is constricted. It can also be demonstrated on a pet: if a dog or cat's head is gently tipped in a backward direction the animal cannot function properly until it re-establishes control over its head, neck and back in relation to each other. This unconscious habit of pulling back the head that so many of us do causes a shortening of the spine and can be a direct cause of many back problems as it can cause an interference of our entire muscular system, which affects our co-ordination, balance and movement.

The primary direction

The first and most important step when starting to give our directions is to ensure a lessening of tension in the neck area so that the natural length of the spine can be restored. The words that you are thinking or imagining must have actual meaning for you, it is not enough just to say the words in a parrot fashion.

The main direction to prevent the habit of pulling the head back is:

1. *Allow the neck to be free*
so that
2. *The head can go forward and upwards*
in order that
3. *The back can lengthen and widen*

Some Alexander teachers may use slight variations of these orders such as:

1. *Allow your neck to be free* is sometimes changed to:

Let the neck be free, or
Think of the neck as being free, or
Think of the neck muscles releasing, or
Think of not stiffening the neck

Alexander himself initially used the order 'relax the neck', but he changed the wording when he found that many of his pupils tended to over-relax their neck muscles.

2.   *The head can go forward and upwards* is often changed to:
Think of allowing the head to go forward and up, or
Let the head go forward and up, or
Allow the head to go forwards and upwards, or
Think of not pulling the head backwards and downwards

3.   *The back can lengthen and widen* can also become:
Think of the back lengthening and widening, or
Allow the back to lengthen and widen, or
Think of not shortening and narrowing the back, or
Let the entire body expand in space

Just use the words which you prefer.

Allow your neck to be free

Notice that the first word is 'allow' – it is something that you let happen and not something you need to achieve. It is unusual for a person to feel this happening, because the majority of the receptors in the neck detect movement rather than tension. These sensory receptors play an essential role in the perception of body orientation and the control of postural alignment. The purpose of this instruction is to eliminate the excessive tension that is almost always present in the muscles of the neck even if we are unable to feel it. It is mainly because it is difficult to feel the release that many people presume that nothing is happening and therefore they 'try to do something' to make it happen, often ending up further away from attaining freedom in the neck than ever before. This is why Alexander lessons are vital as the teacher can tell if you are giving the right instruction. This freedom of the neck joint is essential if your head is ever going to move freely on top of your spine and allow the primary control to perform its natural function. It should always be the first direction given, because unless the primary control is able to organize the rest of the body, any other directions will be relatively ineffective.

It is important to realize what Alexander meant by the neck – he indicated to his pupils that it was high up, away from the shoulders, and situated between the ears, which is the place where the head meets the spine anatomically – known as the atlanto-occipital joint, as it is the connection between the atlas, the top vertebra and the occipital bone of the skull. If you think of this joint becoming free, it will also help neck muscles to become freer as well. I personally have found it very useful to use an actual image, such as the atlanto-occipital joint being filled with oil, both when giving myself directions and when I am teaching others.

So that your head can go forward and upwards

The 'so that' conjunction before this instruction tells you that the two phases are not separate, but are in fact part of the same direction; this part of the instruction determines *in which way* the neck needs to be free. If you just thought of your neck being free without allowing the head to go up, the head may well fall forwards or down or to the side. It is again extremely important that you do not 'do' the direction, but you just allow it to happen as a natural sequence to your neck becoming free. This direction helps to keep the head balanced on top of the spine in such a way that the head goes slightly 'forward' of the spine and the 'up' part of the direction makes sure that the head does not go too far forward. This can help keep the head poised on top of the spine, which keeps it in a state of balance, and it can also help to lead the whole body into a free and flowing movement, because it allows all of the other mechanisms of the body to function naturally and freely. If you think of the head only going forward and not upwards, it would probably drop too far forwards and then

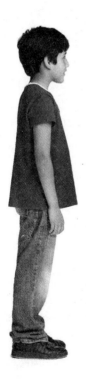

This child has his head naturally going forward and up, and as a consequence his back is lengthened and his muscles are without excessive tension.

downwards as well, causing an increase in muscular tension in the neck area. When you start thinking of the head going up be careful not to pull it back as well, as many people do.

It is important to realize that the forward direction is the head going forward *on the spine* (as if you are about to nod your head affirmatively) and *not* just pushing your face forward. The upward direction of the head is *away from the spine* and not away from the earth, although these may well be the same when the structure is upright. You could imagine that your head is a helium balloon floating upwards and then let your head nod very slightly forwards in an affirming way. A nod that you can just about feel, but no one else can see – you could call it 'an invisible nod'. If you have any confusion about what this instruction means, you may like to pull your head back and down onto the spine for a moment and then stop doing it. When you stop doing it your head will probably go forward and up by itself. I must point out that 'the head forward and up' is a preventative direction that helps to eliminate the usual muscular pull that takes the head back and down, and is in no way a position. In other words, a person can bring their head back in space as they look up at the stars and still have their head going in a forward and up direction. In his book *The Alexander Technique: As I See It*, Patrick Macdonald wrote:

'Forward and up' is not a movement in the accepted sense of the word. It is a tiny extension of the head and spinal column. The movement is so small that it is likely to be seen only by the trained eye, and sometimes not even then. It can, however, usually be readily felt and is none the less real for being small. It is sometimes described as letting the head float off the shoulders. It is something that happens naturally and of its own accord in those few lucky people who are naturally well co-ordinated. It is of the utmost importance that the pupil should not use ordinary muscular means to try and bring this about. It can be achieved by a process of thought or impulse sending.

Later on in the book he adds:

It is useful to consider the 'forward' as an unlocking of the head at the Atlanto-occipital joint by refraining from tightening and pulling it backwards in the accustomary way, and the 'up' as a tiny extension of the spine, which is achieved following this unlocking. The movement, if any, is, in an experienced pupil, so small. It is a directed flow of force or a kind of pulsation, no more than a heartbeat.

Of course, in a badly slumped pupil the lengthening of the spine and the resultant upward movement of the head, while under teacher's manipulation, can be quite extensive, sometimes even adding inches to the pupil's habitual height.

To let your back lengthen and widen

This part of the direction naturally follows the release of the head from the spine and the head moving forward and upwards, and has the effect of reducing the pressure on all the intervertebral discs of the spine. The excessive muscular neck tension which causes the pulling back of the head onto the spine directly causes the spine to shorten, which in turn can put pressure on the discs and literally squeeze them out of place, often putting pressure on the nerves in the back. This direction will help to reverse this and encourage a lengthening of the whole structure. This is invaluable for anyone who suffers with back or neck pain caused by a prolapsed disc. In fact, many people who practise the Alexander Technique can often actually increase in height by 2½cm (1in) or more! The reason a widening direction is included is to prevent the muscles from over-lengthening, which can cause a hollowing in your back while the lengthening of the spine is taking place.

These three parts of the primary directions are in themselves very simple and straightforward. However, some people find them confusing when first practised because they simply involve only thinking of the direction and not 'doing' anything to bring about a change. As I have said before, we have become so accustomed to 'doing' something to help our back pain that it is hard for us to not do anything. Most people are amazed that the solution to what may have been a long-standing back problem could be so simple, particularly when surgery may even have been advised. It is also important to realize that we are used to living in a fast-moving world, and when results do not happen immediately we presume that the method is not working. It is essential to be patient and observant, and realize that changing the habits of a lifetime does take some time.

Secondary directions

There are many secondary directions, too numerous to mention, but they all involve one part of the body moving away from another part. Whereas the main or primary directions can be applied universally, the secondary directions may be applied to certain conditions or ailments. For example, if a person comes to me with rounded shoulders, I may give them an instruction: 'Let your shoulders widen away from each other'; or if someone comes to me with arthritic fingers, I may ask them to: 'Think of your fingers lengthening'. Some people prefer to think or repeat the words to themselves in a meaningful way, while others actually have a three-dimensional image in their head. It entirely depends on what works for you.

Probably the most important secondary direction is: 'Allow your knees to go forward and away from each other'. This instruction is especially useful when walking, bending down and when sitting down and getting up from a chair. All too often people do these activities by pulling the knees together, which invariably puts strain on the legs and lower back. First of all, sit down and stand up slowly in your usual way and see if you can see or feel your knees moving towards each other. Now allow the knees to bend or unbend while you imagine your knees going forward away from your hip-joints, but also the knees gently moving away from each other. You might also like to think of your knees going over the toes, but make sure that your toes are not pointing inwards already.

Here are some examples of secondary directions commonly used in the teaching of the technique:

- 'Think of your shoulders going away from each other' helps to combat rounded shoulders.
- 'Think of your sitting bones releasing onto the chair' helps to prevent sitting up too straight.
- 'Think of your fingers lengthening as the palm of your hand is widening' is a good instruction if you have tension in your hands.
- 'Think of your wrist and your elbow moving away from each other' helps to prevent a shortening in your arms.
- 'Think of your shoulders dropping away from your ears' helps to prevent hunched shoulders.
- 'Think of your elbows dropping downwards' also helps to prevent hunched shoulders.
- 'Think of your legs lengthening' helps to combat shortening of the leg muscles.

- 'Think of your toes lengthening as the sole of your foot widens' is useful for fallen arches or if you have overarched feet.
- 'Think of a lengthening between your feet and your head' can help general posture.
- 'Think of not bracing the knees back' is an excellent order for people with back pain.
- 'Think of not pushing your hips forward' counters the very common habit of leaning back from the waist and is one of the best secondary directions for those with back pain.
- 'Think of lengthening between the navel and the upper part of the chest' can help with a general pulling down in front.
- 'Think of letting your tail-bone drop downwards' helps to let go of tension in your buttock muscles.
- 'Think of your arms dropping from the shoulders' also helps with neck and shoulder tension.
- 'Allow your left shoulder to release away from your right hip' can also help with a general pulling down in the front and with rounded shoulders.
- 'Allow your right shoulder to release away from your left hip' can also can help with a general pulling down in the front and with rounded shoulders.
- 'Think of your torso moving upwards out of your pelvis' can help with a general lengthening of your whole stature.

Please make sure the primary direction *always* precedes any secondary direction that may be given. The words 'think of' may often be substituted by the word 'allow', or 'think of allowing' or 'let', depending on your preference. It might be interesting to see if different words and phrases have different effects on the body. The most important thing to remember at all times is to bring about a change by thinking alone, and not to try and 'do' anything. As I have said repeatedly, when you try to 'do' anything it always increases the muscular tension, which is the very opposite of what you are trying to achieve. Alexander once said: 'Be careful of the printed matter: you may not read it as it is written down.' So it is strongly advisable that when you start giving directions you have some lessons from a trained Alexander teacher to make sure you are not thinking or doing something that may aggravate the situation.

The last type of direction is thinking of directing your body as a whole entity: 'In what direction am I going?' Perhaps you are leaning too far backwards, forwards or to one side. Or perhaps one part of your body is going one way while another is going in the opposite direction. A very common mistake that many people make when learning the Alexander Technique is that they try to put their body into what they think is a correct position, but in reality they need to be doing exactly the opposite; the main principle we need to be aware of is that the head retains a freedom from the rest of the body no matter what we are doing. So please remember when giving yourself these orders or directions that there is no such thing as a correct position. Alexander once said: 'There is no such thing as right position, but there is such a thing as right direction.'

– 9 –

GIVE YOUR BACK A REST

Don't underestimate the value of Doing Nothing

A. A. Milne

'So what do I have to do to start to release tension myself?' is a very common question once someone realizes that tension could be the root cause of their pain. Well the answer is you emphatically must not 'do' anything to release the tension – you have to 'undo' it and *you cannot do an undoing*! As I have said many times before, if you have back pain your muscles have probably been 'doing' far too much for years. Instead you need to learn how to stop doing so much with your muscles – first of all, you have to learn to do nothing at all with your back muscles so that they start to release and begin to lengthen, and this will give you a much better chance to be able to feel when you are tensing and consequently shortening them. Obviously the most efficient way is to start is to have some Alexander lessons, but while you are waiting for your appointment, and between lessons, you can get some relief by lying down in what is known as the semi-supine position. The word supine simply means lying flat on the ground facing upwards, and because your knees are bent it is called the semi-supine or 'active rest' position. I personally found this course of action very effective when I had my own back problem. I've found that after the first few sessions the semi-supine position often brought instant relief to my back, as it has for many people that I have taught over the years. I did it every day between my Alexander lessons and I highly recommend that anyone with back or neck problems do the same. I still find it a very useful resting position even though I have no pain any more. Here is an interesting story which illustrates how effective the semi-supine procedure can be.

Many years ago, when I was first teaching in the UK, a man came to me with a very, very bad back. He had been suffering pain for more than 25 years and he claimed that he had spent over £87,000 on his back problem. He had documented every single pound he had spent. He started to tell me in detail how he had spent the money: over £3,000 on special chairs, almost £4,500 on the physiotherapist, another £7,000 on the chiropractor, £ 10,000 for special equipment to help him get up the stairs at home and so on. During the first lesson I taught him the semi-supine position and at the end of the lesson he asked me: 'Are you trying to tell me that I did not have to spend that £87,000 on my back over all these years and all I really needed to do was to lie down on the floor with a book under my head and bend my knees?' I thought for a minute and then replied that yes, that was exactly what I was saying. He became visibly upset and even a little argumentative, but he agreed to try it out. For one reason or another I was unable to see him for three weeks and when I did he looked quite different. He told me he had not missed a day doing the semi-supine procedure and in fact had found it the most comfortable position for many years. More to the point, he had not suffered any back pain since he had started the procedure either. He continued with his lessons for a number of weeks and he claimed that he felt like a new man and started to perform activities that he hadn't done for many years. This was a wonderful demonstration of the simplicity and power of the semi-supine position.

The semi-supine position

Many people that have come to me with back pain have found that this procedure is very helpful when first learning how to release the muscular tension that is often the fundamental cause of backache and neck problems. It is a very powerful tool that can help to align the spine and release tension throughout the back, neck and shoulders if it is done regularly.

The purpose of this exercise is to detect and release excessive muscular tension throughout the body. It is easier to let go of tension when lying down because gravity is working on the body in a different way than when we are upright, and there are many more points of contact that your body is making with the ground. Simply lie down on a carpeted floor with your knees pointing up towards the ceiling and some paperback books placed underneath your head. The floor should be firm, but not too hard. Do not use a bed, unless you are unable to get down or up from the floor, or only if you find lying on the floor just too uncomfortable.

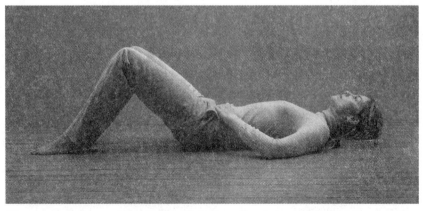

The semi-supine position is one of the best for those people with back pain.

The best way to find the exact height of books to go under your head is to ask your Alexander teacher when you start having lessons, but if there is no teacher near you may follow these instructions:

1. Stand against a flat surface such as a wall.
2. Standing in a relaxed way. Do not try to stand up straight or as though your height was being measured as this will give you false information.
3. Make sure that your heels, buttocks and shoulders are gently touching the wall.
4. Get a friend to measure the distance between the back of your head and the wall – this should be approximately the height of books that you will need.

As a general rule it is better to have too many books than too few. Make sure your head is not so far forward or so far back that it feels uncomfortable, or that your breathing is restricted in any way. Many people find it difficult at first to feel what position their head is in, so it is a good idea to ask a member of your family or a friend to make sure that your head is not tilting backwards, forwards or sideways on the books. If you are still uncertain of the height, it is probably best to use a cushion under your head for the time being until you are able to see an Alexander teacher.

The reason for the books is to encourage the head to release away from the spine so that the spine can lengthen. A lengthened spine is generally much healthier than a shortened one as the discs are under less pressure. If the paperback books feel too hard you may like to place a thin piece of foam or a towel on top of the books so that they feel more comfortable, but as the weeks progress and you are able to release the tension in your neck you may find that you can remove it without any discomfort.

The reason that the knees are bent is so that the muscles in the lower back, which is where many people experience pain, can start to release. Learning to release the tension in the back muscles might take anything from a few days to a few weeks to happen, so please be patient with the process. Many of these tensions have taken years to accumulate – and usually they are not going to disappear overnight. Over time you should feel your back gradually flatten on to the ground, but it is essential that you do not speed up this process by deliberately pushing your back into the ground as this will achieve nothing except even more tension and pain in your back.

As you are lying on the ground you can start to think consciously of releasing the tension in your muscles; you do this by giving your body the directions explained in the previous chapter.

Directions for the semi-supine position

As you are lying on the floor with adequate support under your head make sure your knees are pointing towards the ceiling. The feet should not be too far from the pelvis or too close. Make sure there is no strain in the leg muscles. If the legs tend to fall out, move the feet further apart; if the legs tend to fall in, then move the feet closer together so that the legs are balanced with little effort. Have your hands by your side with the palms of your hands facing downwards or with your hands resting on your abdomen, with the palms facing down. Now merely start thinking the following thoughts and make absolutely sure you are only *imagining* the actions and *not doing anything*. It is better to keep your eyes open, as this is the first step in learning to release tension while you are aware of everything around you. Now you can start to use the following directions.

- Let your neck joint (remember it is situated between your ears) be free in such a way that your head can move slightly forward so that your head can release from the spine (you may like to imagine your nose moving forwards towards your chest a tiny bit).
- Imagine the back of your neck getting longer.
- Imagine your whole spine getting longer (like a telescope lengthening).
- Allow your lower back to spread onto the ground (like butter melting in a frying pan).
- Imagine your two shoulders moving away from one another (like two icebergs drifting apart).
- Imagine your elbows moving away from one another.
- Think of your knees releasing up towards the ceiling.
- Let your feet lengthen and widen onto the ground.
- Imagine that your fingers are lengthening as your palms are widening.

There is little point in thinking these directions just once: you will need to repeat them to yourself over and over again as you are lying on the floor. You may or may not feel any change in your muscles, but even if you don't there may well be some change happening below the level of your conscious awareness. The change that you really want, which is your back pain starting to diminish, may not be felt for some days or even weeks, so please persevere with patience.

Benefits from lying in the semi-supine position

It is important to realize that the following benefits will only arise if this exercise is done on a regular basis (at least once a day for a minimum of 15 minutes) over a period of some weeks. However, do not be overly concerned if you miss the odd day. The best time to lie down is half-way through your day; if this is not always practical, just lie down when you get home from work. Some people find that they have an improved night's sleep if they lie in the semi-supine position just before going to bed; others feel that starting the day in this way suits them better, as they can feel the effects throughout the whole day. It is better not to lie down after a heavy meal, as this will probably feel quite uncomfortable. Make sure you are warm enough, because it is much harder to release tension if you are feeling cold or lying in a draught. If necessary, place a blanket over yourself while you are lying down. You can of course get more benefit if you repeat this procedure two or even three times a day.

When you are horizontal, the back muscles have a greater chance of being at rest and therefore this is the best position in which to release any tension that has built up. When upright, the curves in the spine can sometimes become exaggerated, which can shorten your stature and have detrimental effects on the rest of the body. Being upright is not the problem in itself: it is the way in which we hold ourselves in certain positions while we are on our two feet that puts the spine under so much pressure. Lying down at least once a day can start to alleviate some of this pressure and reduce the muscle tension that has been causing the harmful repercussions in our life. I believe that lying down regularly in the semi-supine position can help to slow down or even reverse the process of deterioration of the bones, discs and joints of the spine. I have seen many cases of rejuvenation of the parts of the body that had suffered from excessive wear and tear caused by an excess of muscle tension.

Here are some of the benefits you may gain by doing the semi-supine position regularly:

- Releases muscular tension throughout your entire body, but especially in the back muscles.

- Reduces pressure on the intervertebral discs.
- Helps to free tension in the neck joint and muscles.
- Lengthens your spine so that it can support you better when you are upright.
- Improves your breathing as you are able to release tension around the ribcage.
- Improves circulation (the blood can flow better through muscles that are relaxed). This also places less strain on the heart.
- You gain a more effective digestion, since the entire system is made up of muscles.
- Frees nerves that have become trapped due to over-tense muscles.
- The internal organs have more room to function.
- Reduces overall stress and tension physically, mentally and emotionally.

Many people have felt that, after doing the semi-supine procedure, they have had more energy in the evening to do the activities that interest them. You may lie in the semi-supine position as many times as you like during the day, but do not stay there for more than 20 minutes at a time. When getting up, do so slowly and mindfully. Do not lift your head off the book and get straight up, but try to roll on to one side as you get up. Try to continue to think about your whole being lengthening as you begin to come back into the standing position. Some people like to listen to instructions on a CD or an MP3 player when doing the semi-supine position and details of these are on the resource page at the end of this book.

Lastly, if at any time you begin to feel uncomfortable while lying down, do not continue with the exercise, simply get up and do it again later. If this uncomfortable feeling continues, please consult your Alexander teacher.

– 10 –

THINKING IN ACTIVITY

Man knows all about the means whereby he can keep the in-animate machine in order, and considers it his duty to make proper use of these, but he knows little or nothing about the means whereby he can keep in order that animate human machine – himself.

F. Matthias Alexander

Alexander was convinced that much of the ill-health that he saw, and which we also see today, was caused by excessive muscular tension. He claimed that a great deal of this tension came directly from what he called the 'habit of end-gaining', which we find in the very fabric of our society today and which often permeates every aspect of our lives. It is natural for us to want to strive to make our lives more comfortable and enjoyable. Yet surely it is just as natural to look at the consequences of the actions as we try to bring about this desired end. We have become so goal orientated that we neglect to pay attention to the way in which we achieve a particular goal. When we fail to do so, we are often heading for trouble. In the simple action of picking up a pen or getting up from a chair we do not give a second's thought to how it is done and we may even become confused when someone suggests that it would be beneficial to pay attention to how we go about our everyday activities, yet it is often during these activities that we do damage to our backs and necks.

It is, of course, necessary for us to have certain goals in life, and to try to attain them is only human. It is what we are doing to ourselves in the process of achieving them that we need to look at. The way we go about our daily activities is a reflection of how we are leading our lives. We need to look after the bodies we live in, and we can do this by performing each action with awareness. We can do this very simply by using the tools of inhibition and direction so that we can consider the course of action at any given movement and develop ways that put our spine and back muscles under the least amount of pressure.

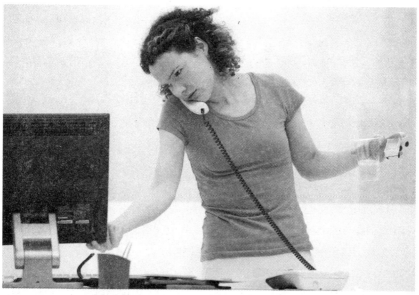

Trying to get a task done, without giving any thought to the best way for that activity to be performed or what we are doing to ourselves has become a habit for many of us.

Trying to get a task done, without giving any thought to the best way for that activity to be performed, has become a habit for many of us – a habit of living for the future rather than being in the present moment. Achieving a goal by considering each step on the way in a conscious manner encourages us to remain in the present, and we are far more likely to achieve the task that we set out to accomplish without doing further damage to our backs and this in turn will give our backs a chance to heal. Attending to the way we perform a task does not mean being over-carefully slow or cautious; it just means applying common sense to any given situation as well as understanding how our body was designed to work.

Trying too hard

Many of us have been encouraged or even taught to try as hard as we possibly can when achieving our goals – in fact it is seen by many as a virtue, although that is not really what life is about. When you think carefully about the way in which actions could be performed more efficiently, you can save yourself a lot of time, effort and discomfort. Alexander disliked the saying 'When at first you don't succeed, try, try, and try again' and apparently had a sign in his teaching room which read: 'When at first you don't succeed, never try again . . . At least not in the same way.' He was convinced that over-trying, over-focusing or concentrating invariably involved excessive and unnecessary tension. This also applies when learning the Alexander Technique: some people try so hard to put the principles into their lives that it is counter-productive. Life is often a lot easier than we make it out to be. When we perform any task, it is essential to inhibit for a moment to really consider the best course of action and this is what Professor John Dewey called 'thinking in activity'. It would be impossible to discuss every action that we do, but let's have a look at some of the most common ones.

Standing

Even when we are just standing still, our bodies are performing an incredible balancing act. We consist of 206 bones and over 650 muscles, which are all inter-relating to one another. Not only that, but we have the weight of the head, approximately 12lb (5.5kg), sitting on top of the spine. All of this makes us extremely unstable, but this instability allows us to make movements with very little effort. If we can release the muscle tension, the reflexes in our body can then organize our extremely unstable structure into an upright posture with little or no conscious effort on our part. However, many of us stand by leaning backwards, forwards or with our weight over to one side, or even only being supported by one leg. Just look around you in a busy shopping street. Most people are completely unaware that they are standing in such awkward ways and that these standing habits can easily lead to back pain. When standing, it is important to have the weight of your body over both feet equally, to make sure that your knees are neither bent nor braced back. When standing for more than a few minutes, it can be helpful to have the feet about 30cm (12in) apart, one foot about 15cm (6in) behind the other, with the feet at an angle of approximately 45 degrees and with slightly more weight on the rear foot – this will give a more stable base that will help the body to maintain an upright posture with the minimum amount of effort. Even if you are leaning backwards, as many people are, standing with one's feet in this position can lessen the pressure on the lower back, as it can help to prevent the common habit of pulling the back in and pushing the pelvis forwards.

Most people are completely unaware that they are standing in such awkward ways and that these standing habits can easily lead to back pain.

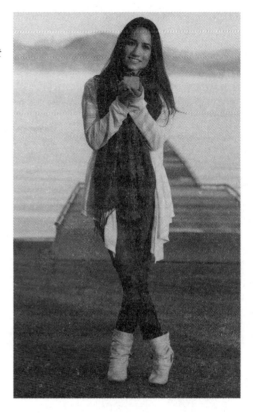

When standing, it is also important to remember the primary directions to allow your neck to be free so that your head can go forward and upwards so that your back can lengthen and widen. You can also help matters by thinking of your feet spreading onto the ground so that the heel, the ball of the foot and the point just below the little toe all have equal contact with the ground. These three points form a tripod and can help to keep us stable while standing. I have found that it is very common for people to have excessive weight on only one or two of these points, which then causes instability throughout the body. When balanced standing is achieved, many muscles throughout the body can begin to release excess tension.

Walking

Just observe a young child and you will see that walking should have a natural easy flow of movement. When children see an object that they want to go towards, their eyes go towards the object of interest. Since their eyes are located in their heads and the weight of the head starts the movement towards wherever they want to go, then the rest of the body simply follows the head. Everything else is organized by the primary control. Many of us, however, are not even looking where we are going, and can easily be lost in our thoughts: this does not give our senses and reflexes a chance to work.

When we bear in mind the principles of inhibition and direction described earlier in the book, walking becomes an action where we are working *with* gravity rather than against it. Walking is a process of releasing certain muscles that support the head on top of the rest of the body, thus allowing the head to move very slightly forward, but in an upwards direction. Since the rest of the body is already in a state of instability, it will then move by slightly falling forwards. As soon as the body detects even the smallest amount of movement the reflex mechanism will automatically and subconsciously bend one knee and send a leg out in front to save the body from falling over. This is all done completely subconsciously. All you have to do is to release the muscular tension that is stopping these reflexes from working perfectly. It is important that you do not try and 'do' this. When practising the Alexander Technique, it is useful to realize that the head always leads any movement and the body naturally follows afterwards.

All other animals, whether it is a mammal, a bird or a fish, move with their heads leading; which is why the main sensory organs (eyes, ears, nose and tongue) are all situated in the head. At first this may seem like an obvious statement, but few of us apply this principle when moving and you can often see the head moving backwards on the spine as the person is moving forwards.

In contrast to children, many adults take a step by lifting the leg with the thigh muscles against the pull of gravity. This expends unnecessary energy and if you think about how many steps you take in one day alone you will realize how much energy is wasted. Not only is there a waste of energy, but also an increase in tension throughout the whole structure simply to maintain balance when one foot is raised from the ground. This tension is perfectly harmless if it is occasional, but when it occurs thousands of times a day it often leads to an overly tense muscular system and eventually this could lead to back pain.

A word about footwear

Dr William Rossi, a doctor of podiatric medicine (DPM) and consulting footwear editor of the *Journal of the American Podiatric Medical Association*, has researched extensively into the effects modern shoes have on health. He states that in shoe-wearing societies a visibly faulty gait can often be corrected and made normal, but it can *never* be made natural as long as conventional shoes are worn. He claims that it is biomechanically impossible because most shoes force an alteration of the foot away from the natural position and by doing so detrimentally affect stance, postural alignment, body balance, equilibrium, body mechanics and weight distribution. The role of shoe heels has been given much attention in the literature because their influence on posture is so obvious, especially with heels of two or more inches in height. Even a one-inch heel throws the body forwards by as much as ten degrees. So with a three-inch heel a person is thrown forward by an incredible 30 degrees. The body tries to rectify itself by leaning back and often does this by overarching the lumbar curve and this in itself can cause a lot of damage to the back.

Dr Rossi points out:

For the body to maintain an erect position, a whole series of joint adjustments in the ankle, knee, hip, spine and neck are required to regain and retain the erect stance. In this reflex adjustment scores of body parts – bones, ligaments and joints, muscles and tendons – head to foot must instantly change position. If these adjustments are sustained over prolonged periods, or by habitual use of higher heels, as is not uncommon, the strains and stresses become chronic, causing or contributing to aches of legs, back and shoulders, fatigue, etc.

People often ask me whether I can recommend a shoe that is good for the feet while walking. The only shoe that I am aware of, which has been designed according to the principles of the Alexander Technique and with Dr Rossi's observations in mind, was actually designed by my son, Tim Brennan, while he was at the Royal College of Art in London, and after having had a series of Alexander lessons. He designed a shoe primarily to help him play tennis without damaging his feet. He called the shoe the Vivo Barefoot Shoe and it is now on sale worldwide. The shoe has no heel and allows the feet and ankle to work freely as nature intended, as it allows the plantar flexion movement of the foot to work without interference, as well as having plenty of room in the shoe for all of the joints of the feet to move freely. Full details of this shoe can be found on the VIVOBAREFOOT website whose address can be found at the back of this book. These shoes are not a substitute for learning the Alexander Technique, but with a combination of Alexander lessons and wearing beneficial footwear that allows one to walk naturally, you will be able to walk and stand with greater ease and with less pain.

Bending and lifting

Back pain often starts or is exacerbated when bending or lifting and this is because this action is usually performed badly. Bending down is an amazing balancing act and needs to be carried out with awareness. When bending down to pick objects up, it is important that one part of the body is counter-balanced with another part, yet many people do not bend in this way. Due to excessive muscle tension it is often the case that adults in industrialized society do not bend their knees, hips or ankle joints. These are the three major joints in the body designed to raise or lower us and if they get underused they will become stiffer and stiffer. You will often see people bending at the waist, where there is actually no hinge joint at all – they are in reality bending their spines. There is an interesting story about some missionaries who went to Africa around 1930 and mixed with some native people. The native people were awestruck by the fact that the white missionaries often bent down from the waist without bending their knees at all (see illustration on page 48). The Africans could not believe their eyes as this way of moving was so alien to them and they adopted a long African name for the white man which when directly translated meant 'the tribe without knees'.

This way of bending may not only cause us to directly damage the spine, it can also cause the body to be completely out of balance, immediately putting enormous strain on the entire muscular system, especially the back and neck muscles, which have to tighten in order to prevent us from falling over. The crucial point here is that, without realizing it, when getting up again after bending people are actually lifting their own body weight with their back muscles every time they bend to pick up even a light object, causing them to use far more effort than is necessary. This sort of misuse is a disaster for the body, and, if habitual, can often directly cause lower-back pain and neck

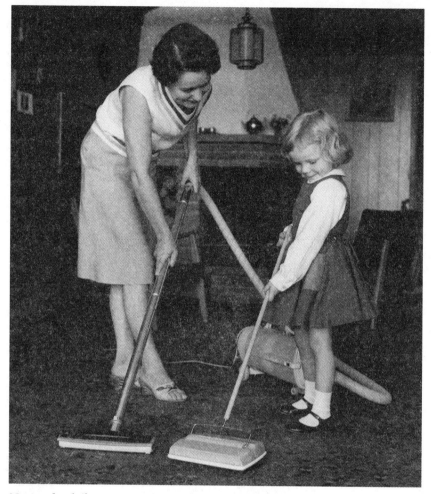

Notice the different ways that children and adults do the same task.

problems. What's more, all the internal organs are put under pressure and breathing is restricted. If you ever watch young children or indigenous people, you will see that they squat when bending, using their very powerful leg muscles rather than their back muscles. You will rarely see young children or indigenous people bending down without bending their hips, knees and ankles (see illustration on page 50). All joints require natural and regular movement to keep them healthy, so by releasing tension and using your major joints naturally in order to maintain balance and equilibrium, you will also be keeping your joints free from problems and your muscles perfectly toned.

Exercise

Try picking a magazine off the coffee table in your usual way, and stop just as your hand reaches it, and ask yourself the following questions: 'Are my knees bending?' 'If so, by how much?' 'Do I feel in balance or unbalanced?' 'Can I feel any tension in my body, and if so, where?' 'How much overall effort am I using in this simple activity?'

Now repeat the same action, only this time make a conscious decision to stop and refrain from your usual habit, this gives you a moment to allow freedom of your neck so that your head can move forward and upwards and your spine can lengthen. At the same time, allow your knees to bend so that they go forward and away from each other. Allow them to bend more than you normally would, but make sure that you are not pulling them in towards one another. Does this feel more balanced and easier on your muscles and joints? You will help yourself to improve overall posture overnight if you start to use the hip, knee and ankle joints as nature intended in order to keep you balanced in the hundreds of actions you perform every day.

Moving from sitting to standing

Many of us make a big deal about getting out of a chair or sofa. This is because many of us try to leave the chair in a vertical fashion, and by doing this we think of ourselves as having to fight gravity, putting enormous strain on our entire structures. But getting out of a chair is simply transferring weight from the pelvis onto the feet and can feel effortless if we use the body's natural mechanisms and reflexes. When getting up, make sure that your feet are a little apart and not too far forward. Each knee should be roughly above the front of the corresponding foot. As you begin to stand up, allow your head to move first by allowing it to go slightly forward and upwards, away from your spine, then allow the rest of your body to follow. Make sure your head does not drop downwards or get pulled back As more weight goes onto your feet you may feel an increased pressure under the feet, which triggers your postural reflex, and this will help you to leave the chair with less effort than usual. As you leave the chair, allow your hip, knees and ankles to 'unbend' rather than straightening your legs or pushing your feet into the floor. When getting up from a sofa make sure you move to the edge of the sofa before trying to get up.

If done in a balanced way you should be able to pause at any moment with grace and ease and feel totally balanced. If in doubt as to what to do, just watch a three year old!

Moving from standing to sitting

A common habit that many of us have is to fall backwards when sitting down. This immediately excites our fear reflexes and causes the head to retract backwards, the shoulders to hunch and the back to overarch as the body subconsciously senses it is off balance and tries to protect itself from falling. Again, if this is the habitual way we sit down, the body will retain this tension unconsciously and the neck, shoulders and back can constantly remain in a state of tension. The natural way to sit down is to allow the head to move slightly forwards without dropping down too much, while at the same time bending the hips, knees and ankle joints so that you descend in perfect balance. Again, you should be able to pause at any moment and be balanced with ease. As your sitting bones reach the chair, allow them to roll back, keeping your head balanced on your spine and your back in a lengthened state. If you are really in balance, you will be able to change your mind and get up any time you want without making any effort.

The same principles apply to any action you perform. If your body is out of balance, your muscles and joints will become tense and stiff and if your body is in balance, your joints and muscles should be free and your movements easy.

It would take too long to look at every movement we make, but the following principles can be applied to working at a computer, driving a car, running and swimming, or to any of the thousands of activities we do.

- Always inhibit your first reaction to give yourself time to think of the most effective and efficient way of performing any given activity.
- Give your directions before and while performing the activity.
- Be aware of any old detrimental habits that might creep back as you are performing the activity.
- Don't be too goal orientated to get the task completed.
- Enjoy the moment.
- Always be prepared to pause again to reconsider or re-choose the way that you are performing your action at any stage.

– 11 –

PSYCHO-PHYSICAL UNITY

You translate everything, whether physical mental, or spiritual, into muscular tension.

F. Matthias Alexander

In this chapter we shall consider the fact that back pain may be caused for mental and emotional reasons. Alexander claimed that we translate everything, whether physical, mental or spiritual, into muscular tension and like the early philosophers he realized that our mind, body and emotions are all intrinsically interconnected. Hippocrates, often referred to as the father of modern medicine, was a firm believer that the healing of the body cannot be separated from the health of mind and emotions. He held the strong view that with the right mental and emotional conditions, the body has a natural ability to heal itself. Today, in so many treatments for back pain, it is the back alone that is examined and treated. However, not only can pain often be referred from different parts of the body, it also can be caused or exacerbated by our mental and emotional states. Back pain may indeed be a 'wake-up call' that is showing us that we need to make fundamental changes to the way we are living.

Back pain and emotions

Different emotions or thoughts can also affect muscle tension: if we feel angry, irritable, depressed or stressed, we will probably be tensing our muscles as well. Next time you are late for an appointment, try to be aware of how much tension you are holding in your shoulders, neck or back; if we are constantly under pressure in our life, this tension will be present continually. During his years of discovery, Alexander realized that the body, mind and emotions did not only affect one another, they were in fact inseparable – he referred to this principle as psycho-physical unity. This fundamental principle of the Alexander Technique, which states that the body, mind and emotions are merely different facets of the same entity, means that if we change one thing we change all of them. It is easy to see this principle all around us: for example, the posture of a tennis player who is walking off the court after losing a match is totally different to the way the same player moves when he has just won a match. The way people stand at a bus stop waiting to go to work at a job that they do not enjoy will be very different from when the same people are just about to go on holiday. What we are thinking and feeling will directly affect the way we sit, stand and move. Since the whole basis of the Alexander Technique rests on the principle of psycho-physical unity, it follows that any physical habits we have will invariably affect our mental and emotional states as well. So if we are able to change the way that we perform our daily activities, our mental attitude to life will also change, and this in turn can alter how we feel emotionally.

It also follows then that feelings of unhappiness or unfulfilment of any kind must directly affect the way we use our physical bodies and this is why Alexander used the term 'the use of the self' and not just the 'use of the body', as the self includes the way we think and feel. In other words, by applying the principles of inhibition and direction to our actions we can also alter the way in which we think and feel, and this can change our life for the better. As you will see from the case histories in chapter fourteen, it was not only people's backs that changed – it was also the way they were living.

No one starts out in life feeling angry, frustrated, lacking in confidence or self-worth: these are habits of thought that we acquire throughout our lives and are not inherent to our mental or emotional make-up. All emotional or mental experiences, whether negative or positive, will affect our muscles accordingly. If these experiences are stressful and happen often enough, then the muscles learn to stay in a state of tension, which eventually becomes habitual. A good example of psycho-physical unity is a person suffering from depression. Although it is a mental illness, sometimes you can actually see the physical depression in their posture. The word depression is also used to describe a physical shape. So often, mental depression can manifest in the shape of the physical body and sometimes changing posture can alleviate despondent thoughts.

Releasing muscular tension throughout the body can sometimes result in releasing emotions, but do not be concerned as this is quite normal and any feelings that may arise will soon pass. As one becomes freer physically, there can also be a corresponding increase in mental and emotional freedom. It is much better, in my opinion, to have these unconscious tensions released rather than being trapped within the body, causing us to behave in detrimental ways both towards ourselves and others. It is important that we release the tension ourselves and learn ways of avoiding tension in the future as this helps us to become empowered to make conscious decisions that can change our lives for the better. It is often the case that a person approaches me purely because of a back or neck problem, yet they often say after a few Alexander lessons that they are feeling calmer, more alert and happier as a result of less muscular tension.

Other people report that they are sleeping better or that their home life is more harmonious, while others are surprised because their confidence and self-esteem has increased.

Stress

One of the biggest emotional factors that contribute to back pain is stress. We are living in the 'age of speed' where, although we are surrounded by a vast range of 'timesaving' technological machines, a great many people still feel they don't have enough time. Back pain and a feeling of rushing from one task to the next are very much connected, as can be seen in common expressions such as being 'pressed for time', 'pushed for time' or 'under pressure of time'. This feeling that we don't have enough time often causes harmful tension throughout the body, but this lack of time is more of a feeling or a thought than a reality. As young children we felt we had all the time in the world, and we were firmly rooted in the present moment. The summer months seemed endless. Young children have little or no concept of time; they do not run because they feel late – they run because they enjoy the feeling of running. This feeling that they have all the time in the world is reflected in their graceful posture and free movements.

As we get older, however, time constraints put on us by school or work commitments cause us to become more and more concerned about the consequences of being late, and we are actively encouraged to be over-concerned for the future, thus being less and less engaged in the present moment. Our lives as adults are commonly filled with appointments for specific times, and if we are late we feel that that may cause trouble, even if we are simply meeting a friend for coffee. These emotional feelings can often manifest as muscular tension, which can cause the vertebrae and discs to be pushed out of place.

We are generally taught that doing things quickly is far better than doing things well and as a consequence many of us feel that every job we undertake has to be done at speed, and yet this takes the enjoyment out of everything we do. Even as far back as 1910, Alexander believed that the human race was becoming increasingly goal orientated, and that this was affecting people's health in a detrimental way. Today this kind of stress has multiplied beyond anything Alexander could have imagined. Have a look at people in the city rushing to get to their destination. Typically their shoulders will be hunched up and pulled forward, their heads will be pulled back and down onto their spines and their backs will be arched. Obviously this can contribute directly to back pain, so a vital step in preventing future back pain is to begin to give ourselves more time in everything we do. Realizing that life is not one long emergency really helps to reduce muscle tension.

The habit of rushing

The habit of rushing from one thing to the next is a problem that not only affects us physically, but it also affects us mentally, emotionally and spiritually. Feeling that we do not have enough time affects us mentally: by over-stimulating the mind, eventually causing mental blocks, an overactive mind that gives us little or no control over persistent unwanted thoughts, and endless worry for no reason. It affects us emotionally, because it can cause us to lose control of our anger and react irrationally, which eventually can damage relationships with family or friends. It can affect us spiritually, because it prevents us from being in contact with the peace and tranquillity that should be the very essence and foundation of our lives. Stress prevents us from 'being human' in the truest sense of the word and turns us into 'doing machines', which in time will start to break down.

At first, we may actively enjoy the buzz of the adrenaline as it rushes around the body when we take on new and exciting challenges, but sustained over a long time, stress can rob us of everything that is important. It can take away our good health and replace it with an aching neck or back, or one of a wide range of other stress-related disorders. Many of us today have forgotten the art of how to be at peace.

Changing the habit of rushing

The first thing to do is to notice how you feel when you are in a hurry. Notice the position of your head and shoulders. See if you can feel tension in other parts of your body, for example, the back, the legs, the arms and even your jaw. Ask yourself how important is it that you get to your destination as quickly as possible. You may realize that there is actually no hurry and that you are rushing out of habit. It is important to differentiate between doing things quickly and rushing our movements: there is nothing wrong with doing things quickly, it is constant hurrying that harms us.

Exercises

1. Lie on the floor with your eyes closed.
2. Think of being in a stressful situation, such as being late for work and you have lost your car keys, and then imagine you get stuck in traffic on the way to work and then finally you get a puncture!
3. See if you can feel a change in the tension in your muscle, your breathing and heartbeat.

Now repeat a different scenario:

1. Again lie on the floor with your eyes closed.
2. This time think of relaxing on a beach or in your garden on a beautiful summer's day. Imagine that you are feeling content and everything feels perfect.
3. After a few minutes see if you can feel a difference in muscle tension.
4. Is your breathing and heartbeat different than before?

Remember it is only your thinking that has changed, but you are probably aware that your thinking has affected your physical and emotional states. This exercise clearly demonstrates how the mind, body and emotions are, in essence, one thing. Sometimes a back problem can be life's way of slowing you down if things have become too frantic and stressed. If you can take stock and use this time to really examine your life, you may find that your backache is a symptom of stress, and if that is the case, try to make some fundamental changes to your life so that you become the master of time and not the other way around.

– 12 –

THE ALEXANDER TECHNIQUE
AND THE MEDICAL WORLD

*When an investigation comes to be made, it will be found that
every single thing we are doing in the work is exactly what is being
done in nature where the conditions are right, the difference being
that we are learning to do it consciously.*

F. Matthias Alexander

There has been a very mixed reaction to the Alexander Technique
in the medical world. In almost all cases, whether a doctor was
supportive of the technique or not often relied on whether he, or she,
had personally experienced the technique themselves. Even from the
very beginning, the doctors who had Alexander lessons themselves
were often amazed and astounded by its remarkable effects and
would often recommend it highly to their patients. However, from
a distance, without direct experience of the technique, it is very
difficult to understand how it works. This can irritate some scientists
and medical practitioners and they sometimes, even today, come to
the conclusion that the technique is just some inexplicable quackery
or perhaps a form of strange hypnotism. Even when Alexander first
arrived in London with his letters of reference from the Australian

doctors, he was not exactly welcomed with open arms. He was, in fact, greeted with a degree of suspicion by many doctors: they just could not understand how a man, who had never set a foot inside a university, let alone a medical school, could claim that he had discovered a way of helping such a wide range of illnesses with one single technique when many learned people in the medical world were still struggling to find solutions for many of them. Yet even today, many medical researchers are at a loss as to the actual cause of so many back problems. My father, who was an excellent doctor himself, used to say: 'If you want a day off work, you should just say you have back problems, because nobody can prove you have, and nobody can prove you haven't, and even if you have a back problem, nobody can do anything about it.' And it is more or less the same today.

Prior to 1904, while Alexander was still in Australia, several doctors became convinced that Alexander's work was indeed effective, either from their own personal experience or from seeing the effects that the technique had on their patients. These doctors began referring more and more of their patients to Alexander and he started to gain an excellent reputation for helping to cure many conditions previously considered incurable. He used the gentle guidance of his hands, as well as verbal instructions, to convey this new knowledge; many people found this preferable to medication or manipulation, which often had harmful side-effects. He helped more and more people to change the harmful habits that were at the root of their illnesses, and began to recruit other members of his family to help him with his work, in particular his brother, Albert Redden Alexander.

A group of doctors, led by Dr J. W. Stewart McKay, a prominent Sydney surgeon, were so convinced about the importance of Alexander's discovery for the whole of humanity that they persuaded Alexander to go to London to present his work to a much wider audience. So in the spring of 1904 Alexander set sail for London, together with letters of recommendation from several distinguished doctors, and prepared himself to give lectures and talks about his amazing discovery of the primary control.

Early years in London

When Alexander arrived in London in 1904, he was not deterred by his cool reception from the medical profession. He was not put off that some doctors even thought of him as a charlatan or as a complete fraud or con man. As Louise Morgan describes in her book *Inside Yourself*, which was first published in 1954:

[Alexander] observed in every street the results of this wrong manner of use: crooked shoulders, sunken chests, twisted necks, protruding stomachs, swollen joints, blotchy complexions, stiff knees, hobbling legs, bow legs, and doubled over bodies. He saw also in the depressed expressions of faces that deterioration of brain which he knew went hand-in-hand with deterioration of body. In his walks through London he was determined to give his new knowledge to the medical profession for the benefit of these and other sufferers.

The seat of their trouble was *inside themselves*, and could not be cured by drugs, medicines, diet, or any other treatment which came from outside themselves. Their diseases were symptoms indicating the way they managed themselves. If their symptoms were cured, they would probably turn up again in more severe forms in another part of the body. Until the sufferers themselves understood what was happening inside themselves, and changed their old use of themselves to a new one, they would never get really well or know that true happiness of being alive.

Alexander was not in the least dissuaded from his task and he soon obtained some fine clothes, a butler and an impressive address at the Army & Navy Mansions in Victoria Street, central London to work from. In those days, you just couldn't get on in London unless you presented yourself in the right way and it was not long before it was 'business as usual' as he started teaching the people of London. He soon gained supporters within the London medical community, especially from an ear, nose and throat surgeon by the name of R. H. Scanes Spicer, who took lessons himself and personally promoted Alexander's method as well as referring many of his own patients to Alexander.

Over time, more and more doctors became convinced that Alexander had made an all-important discovery regarding the key to good health, including Dr Peter Macdonald, who was chairman of the Yorkshire branch of the British Medical Association. In his inaugural address he publically declared:

Alexander is a teacher pure and simple. He does not profess to treat disease at all. If the manifestations of disease disappear in the process of education, well and good; if not, the education of itself will have been worthwhile. Manifestations of disease, however, do disappear. Including myself, I know many of his pupils, some of them, like myself, are medical men. I have investigated some of these cases, and I am talking about what I know.

He went on to say that although the technique was practically unknown to many doctors, it was of such importance that he declared that an immediate investigation by the medical profession was imperative.

Around this time two senior surgeons in the London hospitals, Andrew Rugg-Gunn, and James E. R. McDonagh, became loyal supporters of the technique and spoke out in favour of Alexander. Rugg-Gunn declared: 'Mr Alexander is an educationist, and not a "healer" or physical culturist. His teaching embodies with complete precision those principles of psycho-biological behaviour, which are among the most recent deductions of experimental physiology, and applies them in man to a constructive art of living.' McDonagh, after meeting Alexander and watching him at work, wrote: 'It became apparent to me that the wrong use of the body plays an important role in disease.'

During the 1930s Sir Charles Sherrington, OM, GBE, PRS, the internationally famous neurophysiologist, who received the Nobel Prize in physiology and medicine in 1932, also became a supporter of Alexander and drew encouraging attention to the technique, stating:

> Mr. Alexander has done a service to the subject [of the study of reflex and voluntary movement] by insistently treating each act as involving the whole integrated individual, the whole psychophysical man. To take a step is an affair, not of this or that limb solely, but of the total neuromuscular activity of the moment, not least of the head and neck.

Around the same time the award-winning anatomist, Professor George E. Coghill, also started to take lessons from Alexander. He was so impressed with the results that he himself achieved that he wrote a six-page introduction to Alexander's book *The Universal Constant in Living*. In it he said:

> [Alexander] seeks to restore the functions of the body through their natural uses. His methods of doing this are original and unique, based as they are on many years of experience and exhaustive study.

Yet they can scarcely be adequately described although the results are marvellous . . . It is my opinion that habitual use of improper reflex mechanism in sitting, standing, and walking introduces conflict in the nervous system, and that this conflict is the cause of fatigue and nervous strain, which bring many ills in their train . . . Mr. Alexander's method lays hold of the individual as a whole, as a self-vitalizing agent. He reconditions and re-educates the reflex mechanisms and brings their habits into normal relation with the functioning of the organism as a whole. I regard this method as thoroughly scientific and educationally sound.

In 1937 a group of doctors, led by Peter Macdonald, wrote a letter to the editor of the *British Medical Journal*. It was signed by no fewer than 19 doctors and stated:

As the medical men concerned we have observed the beneficial changes in use and functioning which have been brought about by the employment of Alexander's technique in the patients we have sent to him for help – even in the case of so called 'chronic disease' – whilst those of us that have been his pupils have personally experienced equally beneficial results. We are convinced that an unsatisfactory manner of use, by interfering with general functioning, constitutes a predisposing cause of disorder and disease, and that diagnosis of a patient's troubles must remain incomplete unless the medical man when making his diagnosis takes into consideration the influence of use upon functioning . . . Unfortunately, those responsible for the selection of subjects to be studied by medical students have not yet investigated the new field of knowledge and experience which has been opened up through Alexander's work, otherwise we believe that ere [before] now the training necessary for acquiring this knowledge would have been included in the medical curriculum. To this end we beg to urge that as soon as possible steps should be taken for an investigation of Alexander's work and Technique . . .

Dr Wilfred Barlow

Unfortunately, due to the outbreak of the Second World War in 1939, all follow-up to this letter was abandoned. However, the first medical research into the Alexander Technique was conducted in the early 1940s by Dr Wilfred Barlow, MD. Dr Barlow was a consultant rheumatologist based at Guy's Hospital in London who was so inspired with his own personal experience of the Alexander Technique that he trained for three years to be an Alexander teacher. His research involved photographing a person before and after Alexander lessons, standing in front of a grid. The grid helped to measure the dramatic postural changes that took place. Another part of his research involved using an electrical device that recorded activity in neck muscles before and after Alexander re-education. He was able to prove that there was far less activity in the neck muscles after a course of Alexander lessons. A good summary of Dr Barlow's research can be found in his book, *The Alexander Principle*, in which he points out that, at the time of writing, to his amazement as a medical doctor, all the Alexander teachers without exception had a clean bill of health: no heart disease, no cancers, no strokes, no rheumatoid arthritis, no disc problems, no ulcers, no neurological disorders. He goes on to say that this was a standard of day-to-day health and happiness that most people encounter only in their earliest years. 'This statistic is almost unbelievable. The gold brick is too good to be true, but it is in fact true, and it is not insufferable arrogance to say that this principle is a must. It is also a plain brute fact that over 99% of the population need it, but know nothing of it.'

Professor Frank Pierce Jones

It was also around the same time (1938) that another man, who was to research extensively into the Alexander Technique, approached Alexander's brother, Albert Redden Alexander, for help. This man was Professor Frank Pierce Jones of Brown University, in the USA, who was continually plagued with fatigue and muscular aches and pains. This is how Professor Jones described his first lesson in his book *Freedom to Change*:

My first experience of making a habitual movement without habitual effort seems as vivid to me now as it was when A. R. Alexander demonstrated the technique to me in 1938. Perhaps it was the element of surprise that made the experience so memorable. I had expected something quite different – to have my faults of breathing and voice production diagnosed and to be given a set of exercises to correct them. Instead, Alexander chose the movement from sitting to standing for his demonstration. He made a few slight changes in the way I was sitting (they seemed quite arbitrary to me and I could not remember afterwards what they were), then asking me to leave my head as it was, he initiated the upward movement without further instructions. Before I had a chance to organize my habitual response, the movement was completed and I found myself standing in a position that felt strangely comfortable. I was fully conscious throughout the movement, and it was a consciousness, not of being moved by somebody else – Alexander appeared to be making no effort whatever – but by a set of reflexes whose operation I knew nothing about.

In addition to the reflex effect, the movement was notable for the way time and space were perceived. Though it took less time than usual to complete the movement, the rate at which they moved seemed paradoxically slower and more controlled and the trajectories that my head and trunk followed were unfamiliar. The impression was that of a sudden expansion in both dimensions, so that more time and space were available for the movement. The most striking aspect of the movement, however, was the sensory effect of lightness that it induced. That feeling had not been present at the start, nor had it been suggested to me; it was clearly a direct effect of the movement. While it lasted, everything I did, including breathing, became easier. After a short time the effects faded away, leaving me, however, with the certainty I had glimpsed a new world of experience which has more to offer than the limited set of movement patterns, attitudes and responses to which I was accustomed.

It was due to the sensory experience of that first lesson that Professor Jones became fascinated with what had caused that lightness of being, physically, mentally and emotionally – one of the hallmarks of the Alexander Technique. Professor Jones dedicated much of the rest of his life to scientifically explaining and verifying the underlying basis for the obvious beneficial effects of having Alexander lessons, and the research that he did at Tufts University in the US took almost three decades to complete. Professor Jones did many studies attempting to scientifically explain how and why the Alexander Technique produces the results that it does. During his extensive research he used multi-image photography, electromyography, force plates and X-ray photography, publishing over 30 papers. During that time, he also corresponded with teachers, scientists, and doctors all over the world, and collected a large body of research data. The result was an extensive and fascinating record of the Alexander Technique. These studies showed that the Alexander Technique could produce a marked reduction in the stress on muscles. His results are included in his book *Freedom to Change: The Development and Science of the Alexander*

Technique and *Collected Writings on the Alexander Technique* and are also documented at the Dimon Institute, in New York City.

Professor Nikolaas Tinbergen

While Professor Jones was writing his book, back in Oxford in 1973, Professor Nikolaas Tinbergen was awarded the Nobel Prize for medicine and physiology. Professor Tinbergen had just had a course of Alexander Technique lessons from Dick and Elisabeth Walker and was so impressed with the results of his lessons that he devoted nearly half of his Nobel Prize acceptance speech to Alexander's work, stating:

> This story of perceptiveness, of intelligence, and of persistence shown by a man without any medical training, is one of the true epics of medical research and practice . . . we already notice, with growing amazement, very striking improvements in such diverse things as high blood pressure, breathing, depth of sleep, overall cheerfulness and mental alertness, resilience against outside pressures, and also in such a refined skill as playing a stringed instrument. So from personal experience, we can already confirm some of the seemingly fantastic claims made by Alexander and his followers, namely that many types of under-performance and even ailments, both mental and physical, can be alleviated, sometimes to a surprising extent, by teaching the body musculature to function differently . . . Although no one would claim that the Alexander treatment is a cure-all in every case, there can be no doubt that it often does have profound and beneficial effects – and, I repeat once more, both in the 'mental' and 'somatic' sphere.

Dr David Garlick

In Australia, the story was similar: a comprehensive series of studies of the underlying physiological mechanisms of the technique was also conducted by Dr David Garlick of the University of New South Wales. After completing his research in November 1998, Dr Garlick wrote an open letter to all of his doctors:

Dear Doctor,

The Alexander Technique can be described as a psycho-somatic, re-educative technique that does not set out to be curative but it may, in fact, have useful effects on musculoskeletal and psychological states.

Alexander's observations pointed out that the brain is designed to control the musculoskeletal system at a subconscious level, allowing the person to direct her/his attention to a variety of other stimuli. The problem for the upright human is that a variety of muscle strategies may become employed, in regard to being upright and in carrying out movements, that are inappropriate – for instance: over contracted muscles around neck, shoulders, buttocks, thighs etc and under contracted postural muscles such as in the lumbar region.

Such problems lay the basis for a range of chronic musculoskeletal dysfunctions-tension headaches, neck problems, breathing problems, low back problems, over-use/repetitive strain problems etc.

Alexander made insightful observations on how a person's attention can be directed to the state of her/his muscles (developing the proprioceptive sense, the 6th sense), learning how to begin to stop inappropriate muscle strategies (termed 'inhibition' by Alexander) and how to lay the basis for easier, reflex responses to gravity that result in effective strategies for being upright and for undertaking movements. For this process of allowing better strategies to develop in the person, Alexander developed a set of 'directions' related to the neck being free or relaxed, the head in a direction of 'forward and up' and the back 'lengthening and widening'.

This learning process, greatly assisted with the skilled hands of a teacher of the Technique, is of value to any individual as well as benefiting those with a range of musculoskeletal and stress-induced conditions.

It is interesting that the Technique has attracted the interest and support of a wide range of eminent people including John Dewey, America's leading educational and scientific philosopher; Sir Charles Sherrington, Nobel Laureate in Physiology/Medicine in 1932; Niko Tinbergen, Nobel Laureate in Physiology/Medicine in 1973.

I have undertaken research into some aspects of the Technique and have referred to these in my booklet: *The Lost Sixth Sense; a medical scientist looks at the Alexander Technique.*

Yours sincerely,

Dr. D Garlick,

Director of Sports Medicine Programs

University of New South Wales

School of Physiology and Pharmacology

ATEAM research

At around the turn of the century another event took place in the south of England that was to change the way that doctors viewed the Alexander Technique. The wife of Professor Paul Little developed significant functional back pain during her thirties. Professor Little had heard of the Alexander Technique and encouraged her to have some lessons. Encouraged by the fact that the technique made a significant difference to his wife's back pain, Professor Little proposed a major research trial to the NHS to observe the effects of the Alexander Technique in helping to reduce or eliminate back pain, and this became known as the randomized controlled trial of Alexander Technique lessons, exercise, and massage (ATEAM). It has been the most significant and extensive research ever carried out in connection with the Alexander Technique and its primary aim was to evaluate the effects of Alexander Technique lessons, exercise and massage on chronic and recurring back pain. The multicentre clinical trial was funded by the Medical Research Council and NHS Research and Development Fund and was led by researcher Professor Paul Little, University of Southampton, and Professor Debbie Sharp of Bristol University; the results were published in the *British Medical Journal* in 2008, which made news around the world.

The trial took nearly a decade to complete, as a total of 579 patients, with chronic and recurrent non-specific low-back pain, were recruited from 64 general practices and were randomly allocated to four different groups. The first group had 6 Alexander Technique lessons, the second group had 24 Alexander Technique lessons, another had 6 sessions of therapeutic massage and the last was a control group. All patients continued to receive usual GP care during the trial. Half the participants also received a GP prescription for general exercise with behavioural counselling from a practice nurse. All participants in the Alexander Technique groups were taught by experienced Alexander teachers, who were all registered with the Society of Teachers of the Alexander Technique (STAT). All the Alexander teachers had undertaken a three-year full-time course consisting of at least 1,600 hours of class work. These teachers used hand contact, together with verbal explanation and advice, to increase the participants' awareness of their postural support and movement patterns. During the trial the two main self-reported outcome measures that were used were:

a) the Roland Morris disability score: the 'industry standard' outcome measure for back function

b) days in pain in the past four weeks

Ten other outcome measures were also used. The results of the trial clearly demonstrated that taking one-to-one lessons in the Alexander Technique led to a *long-term* reduction in back pain. In the group which had 24 lessons the average number of days in pain was three days per month, compared with an average of 21 days per month for people in the control group; this was an impressive 86 per cent reduction in pain. One year after the trial started, significant improvements were reported in function and quality of life by those who had had 24 lessons, with a 42 per cent reduction in the Roland Morris disability score compared with the control group. Out of all the approaches tested, the group that had 24 Alexander lessons received the most benefit.

Interestingly, the effect of massage on the Roland Morris score was no longer significant after one year, while the effect of Alexander lessons was maintained and patients still continued to report improvement one year after the trial began. The trial authors concluded that the long-term benefits of taking lessons are unlikely to be due to placebo effects of attention and touch and more likely to be due to active learning and application of the Alexander Technique in daily life. Finally, reassuringly, there were no adverse effects whatsoever reported in the trial by any of the 288 participants in the Alexander Technique groups.

Despite this extensive and highly regarded research, which categorically shows that lessons in the Alexander Technique can give *long-term* relief to those suffering with back pain, there are still comparatively few doctors who would refer their patents to an Alexander teacher for various reasons. First of all, very few doctors have had any training in, or awareness of, the Alexander Technique, and they generally include it with all the other alternative or complementary therapies, despite the fact that it is educational and is not a therapy at all. If they do have any awareness of the existence of the technique, they think of it as a 'posture-improving technique which they think should be the job of physiotherapists anyway'. Second, referral into the private sector has historically been an issue of conflict for some traditional doctors, fearing that they may suffer repercussions if a treatment they recommend causes problems. The fact that the Alexander Technique is very gentle, non-invasive, has no side effects – no one to my knowledge has ever reported any adverse effects in over 100 years – is not taken into account. Thirdly, despite the fact that back pain is on the increase and 80 per cent of the population suffer with it, the common medical view that back pain is a self-limiting condition still remains, a condition that is best self-managed with activity and exercises, and therefore physiotherapy and orthopaedics still dominate opinion on medical management of back pain. Lastly, there is still an underlying feeling amongst those involved with traditional medicine that to refer a patient to a non-medical method would be 'selling out' or 'going over to the other side'.

Despite all these setbacks, the Alexander Technique is slowly becoming better known and a growing number of doctors in recent years are beginning to confidently refer some of their patients to Alexander teachers, and in fact in the UK lessons in the technique may now be covered by the National Health Service.

Research with surgeons

Even more recently there was a very interesting pilot study, where medical surgeons themselves took part in the research; the object of the trial was to examine the impact of the Alexander Technique in improving posture and surgical ergonomics during minimally invasive surgery (MIS)

The study was conducted during 2009 and 2010 at the Cincinnati Children's Hospital Medical Center, where seven urologists were given an eight-day intensive course of Alexander Technique lessons; these were taught by Jennifer Roig-Francolí and Lois Cone, both Alexander certified by the American Society for the Alexander Technique (AmSAT). The aim of the study was to discover whether training in at the technique could help improve the surgeons' posture and co-ordination while performing laparoscopic surgical procedures.

'The goal of our research is to prove beyond doubt that this technique works to improve surgical ergonomics and proficiency so that it can be incorporated as part of graduate surgical training,' said Dr Pramod P. Reddy, MD, lead investigator and director of pediatric urology at Cincinnati Children's Hospital. 'Minimally invasive procedures require surgeons and assistants to maintain awkward, non-neutral and static postures of the trunk and extremities. This limits the natural shifting of their posture and can lead to discomfort, fatigue and even injury.'

The subjects were tested in many different areas before and after the training. The results of the training program showed statistically significant improvements in overall posture and specifically upper body and shoulder endurance. Without exception all the surgeons experienced subjective improvement in their overall posture and a definite reduction in discomfort while performing MIS manoeuvres. The study clearly showed that further research is warranted as it points to the possibility that Alexander Technique training for surgeons could help reduce surgical errors related to surgical fatigue syndrome and also reduce the number of repetitive stress injuries to which MIS surgeons are prone. The research was so successful from the surgeons' point of view that it was published in the *Journal of Urology* in 2011, and was presented at two major US medical conferences in 2010; it won second prize for clinical research papers at the national conference of the American Academy of Pediatrics in 2010.

In recent times more and more doctors are standing up and publicly praising the Alexander Technique, as you can see from the following examples:

The Alexander Technique stresses unification in an era of greater and greater medical specialization. Its educational system teaches people how to best use their bodies in ordinary action to avoid or reduce unnecessary stress and pain. It enables clients to get better faster and stay better longer. This is undoubtedly the best way to take care of the back and alleviate back pain.

Dr Jack Stern, spinal neurosurgeon and founding partner
of Brain and Spine Surgeons of New York

The Alexander Technique remains the best of the self-care strategies to prevent the sequel of poor posture and poor breathing.

Dr Harold Wise, MD, PC, New York, NY

Lessons in the Alexander Technique taught me how to sit in a state of lumbrosacral poise, and my chronic low back pain gradually became cured. The Technique is true education. Compared to surgery (e.g. for low back pain or for chronic obstructive lung disease) a course of instruction is inexpensive.

Dr John H. M. Austin, MD, Professor of Radiology;
Chief, Division of Radiology,
Columbia-Presbyterian Medical Center,
New York, NY

The Alexander Technique makes sense in that appropriate use of the body will lead to reduction of various musculoskeletal disorders and remediate others which are established. No equipment is needed, just the skill and training of the teacher. This technique is very worthwhile as a primary preventative therapy. It is especially useful when posture is a key factor in back injuries while lifting and for workers who perform repetitive tasks while sitting.

Dr Robert D. Greene, MD, Emergency Department,
Norwalk Hospital, Norwalk, CT

I recommend people to the Alexander Technique who have not improved with traditional rehabilitative therapies. Part of their pain may be due to posture and the improper use of their bodies. Many people who have neck or back pain and have gone through heat, ultrasound and massage with no relief can be helped by learning the Alexander Technique. It definitely works. Nothing works for everyone; as one well-versed in using physical therapy and biofeedback, I know how valuable this technique is. I highly recommend it.

Dr Barry M. Schienfeld, MD, Specialist in Rehabilitation Medicine
and Pain Management, Community General Hospital, Harris, NY

The Alexander Technique can help relieve pain and prevent recurrences by correcting poor posture and teaching proper patterns of movement.

Dr Andrew Weil, MD, American physician and author
of many books, including *Health and Healing*

A few years ago, Dr Kieran Tobin, a medical consultant, came to see me because of an ongoing neck problem; he was consultant surgeon at the University College Hospital in Galway, Ireland and had been the president of both the Irish Otolaryngological, Head and

Neck Society and the ENT Section of the Royal Society of Medicine of Ireland. He had also been involved in teaching the medical students during their training to be doctors. He was kind enough to write a short appraisal for my last book *Change Your Posture, Change Your Life*. This is what he wrote:

> Neck problems are virtually an occupational hazard for Ear, Nose and Throat surgeons. I had serious problems during my working years, but hoped for relief on early retirement. This was not the case and limitation of cervical (and thoracic) movement became quite an intrusion on my life. Physiotherapy and medication gave only short-term improvement. On being introduced to the Alexander Technique I was somewhat sceptical that anything was going to work, but can only describe the relief gained, and maintained, as quite incredible. General posture has improved and neck mobility has returned to that last experienced more than twenty years ago. What more could one ask for?

In fact Dr Tobin was so impressed with the results of the Alexander Technique that when interviewed by the *Irish Times* he said that he thought that medical students should certainly be made aware of the technique during their training.

– 13 –

THE ALEXANDER EXPERIENCE

Experience is not what happens to a man. It is what a man does with what happens to him.

Aldous Huxley

It is a very difficult task to get someone to understand any experience that they have never had themselves. Try explaining to an Eskimo who has never tasted Indian food what an onion bhaji tastes like, or try to describe what a lychee tastes like to a child who has never tasted one, or what a sunrise looks like to someone who has been blind from birth. It is a similar problem with the Alexander Technique, because in essence it is an experience and that is exactly why it is so hard to explain to others. Even the great writer Aldous Huxley was very reticent about describing the kinaesthetic effect that he had had during his Alexander lessons and argued that it was impossible to impart a sensory experience to someone who has not had it himself. 'It would be', says Huxley, 'like describing the colour red to someone who was colour blind.'

During his research into the Alexander Technique, Professor Frank Pierce Jones asked his subjects to write down their experience in words after having an Alexander lesson. His subjects often reported that their movements felt easier and smoother and they felt lighter and taller while performing simple actions such as walking or bending. Others described it with phrases like: 'More ease and lightness', 'a feeling of ease or competence – very different from "relaxation"' or 'a greater degree of ease and consequent pleasure'. In his book *Freedom to Change*, he writes:

> The feeling of pleasure in everyday movement takes those subjects by surprise, and their faces break spontaneously into a smile as they notice it. 'It's a funny thing,' one of them said. 'It's as if my arms like moving this way and wanted to do it again.' To some subjects the idea of moving against gravity (as in getting up from a chair) without effort is difficult to grasp 'a sense of wonderment'. In describing the experience one said: 'First I was sitting down, and then I were standing up. I don't know how I got there – the movement seemed absolutely impossible.' Another reported, 'Until you had performed it, when it was unbelievably simple – like walking straight into a wall only to find when you have reached it that there was no wall and you will pass through into the space beyond.'

Describing the technique

Other people over the years have tried to describe the feeling that the Alexander Technique imparts: John Cleese, the famous comedian and actor also said the same kind of thing: 'I find the Alexander Technique very helpful in my work. Things happen without you trying. They get to be light and relaxed. You must get an Alexander teacher to show it to you.' Edward Maisel, director of the American Fitness Research Institute and consultant to the President's Council on Physical Fitness, also found lessons in the Alexander Technique extremely effective. In his book, *The Resurrection of the Body*, he described the benefits of these lessons:

> There are an overall flexibility and tonic ease of movement, greater freedom in the action of the eyes, less tension in the jaws, more relaxation in the tongue and throat, and deeper breathing because of the effect of the new alignment on the diaphragm. There is also a sense of weightlessness and a diminution of the effort previously thought necessary to move one's limbs. Activity is now more free and flowing – no longer jerky and heavy with strain.

After his own research about the technique, Dr Chris Stevens concluded in his book *The Alexander Technique*:

> The Alexander Technique appears to progressively release the body from habitual attitudes, perhaps by facilitating righting reflexes. This in turn starts the process of bringing the body into a natural upright posture characterised by greater height, greater shoulder and chest width, and better balance. Also noted are faster and less effortful movement patterns, improved responses to stress, greater respiratory, circulatory and digestive efficiency, and improvements in performance. It appears to improve proprioceptive acuity thus aiding the learning of skills.

Máirtín O'Connor, leading traditional Irish accordion player, had a unique way of expressing the feeling that he experienced:

> After an Alexander session it felt like someone had poured a full canister of three-in-one oil into my neck. After two sessions, I felt 20 years of neck tension fade away and I felt my chest naturally expand. I used to wrap myself round my instrument for years and when your

head is inside the music, it's like an anaesthetic, you don't feel the discomfort, but I gradually became aware of how I had been causing myself problems. I feel I have a greater sense of control when I'm playing if I consciously relax and it's easier overall, particularly if I'm playing something that is technically difficult.

To this day, I remember the feeling I had after my first Alexander Technique lesson. It was totally unique and very, very different from all the other things I had tried. Like Professor Jones, it also took me completely by surprise. I felt taller, lighter, more spacious and my arms and legs felt longer; all my movements became less effortful and it really was like I was walking on air, even though, paradoxically, I had more of a sense of the ground at the same time. In fact, I was so surprised that it took me a while to realize I was no longer in pain! But there were other things too. I felt a great sense of peace, both mentally and emotionally. It felt as though someone had turned off a radio in my head that had been constantly on for many years: my chattering mind had been silenced, but I did not know how. When I was 19 I had learned to meditate and on a few occasions I had completed an eight-hour 'all night' meditation that imparted a feeling of great serenity at the end of it while watching the sunrise. This experience was very similar, but the teacher, to my mind, had hardly done anything and it all happened within 30 minutes. This mental peace that I felt was also accompanied by an emotional calmness; it was like the feeling of watching a very still lake in the evening time: a feeling that everything was in its right place and all was well with the world.

As you can probably understand this would hardly be a satisfying explanation about what actually happened for a medical or scientific person; it was as though the reduction of back pain was a by-product of the connectedness of my mind, body and spirit. I was, for the first time for ages, in harmony with myself. My mind, body and emotions were working in harmony together instead of continually being disconnected from each other. I felt that I had arrived at the present moment instead of constantly trying to be ahead of myself.

The Champagne feeling

Even today, lessons that I have produce similar experiences, but they have not been as surprising as the first time for two reasons. First of all, the tension in my muscles is less now than when I had my original lesson so when I now release tension these days the contrast is not so great, and secondly, my mind now knows what to expect. After a few lessons I was able, to a certain extent, to learn to detect and release some of the muscular tension for myself by using the semi-supine position, as well as being more conscious about how I go about my daily activities. I also noticed that even my breathing became less strained and life in general was much less of an effort. I began to notice that my everyday life became more of a flow and much less of a struggle. After a month or so, I began to notice how restless my mind was, constantly telling me I was not good enough or that this or that was wrong with my life. Over time, practising the technique seemed to help me quieten my mind, and the more peaceful I felt, the more I could see how much out of control my thoughts had been and how much I was constantly reacting to my own thoughts.

I began to see clearly that there was a definite correlation between the amount of mental activity that was going on in my head and how tense my back muscles were. I still have Alexander lessons today, not because of any back pain, but because there is always something I can learn about myself that can improve the quality of my life and consequently the lives of those around me. One of my pupils once said to me that since he started to have Alexander lessons everyone around him at home had changed for the better. The family, however, were adamant that the only change that had happened was within the man, who had become much more pleasant to live with. Even in business meetings and other social situations, the atmosphere can be much more harmonious and efficient if those participating are calmer. When working in companies I have certainly found that people are able to think more clearly and as a result can be more creative with their ideas after a course of Alexander lessons.

The experience of the Alexander Technique actually puts you in touch with your own true essence, an experience that some people may not have had since childhood. It can give us the power to alter our consciousness, which can allow spontaneous gratitude to take the place of negative thinking; since our consciousness has no limits, there is no end to how attentive or appreciative we can be of this amazing existence. The more aware we are, the more alive we will feel and the greater our capacity to enjoy life will be. As the process of change starts to take place, back pain, fear and worry simply evaporate by themselves. One of my earliest pupils called the experience she had after each lesson the 'champagne feeling'. I asked her what she meant and she said 'I feel so light and bubbly with joy after every lesson.' I had another pupil who came to me with back problems and over time many of her friends and relatives came to me for lessons. I became so curious that one day I asked her: 'What do you say to encourage so many people to come for lessons.' She replied: 'When people ask me what the Alexander Technique is, I just say I can't explain it and if you really want to know you will have to go and experience it for yourself. So they all come purely out of curiosity as to why I am so much better than I was.'

Obviously different people will have different experiences of the technique, but the vast majority of people I teach do feel lighter, have an overall feeling that their movements are freer and easier or that their joints have been well oiled as a result of letting go of muscular tension. For some, this kinaesthetic lightness is felt immediately after the first lesson; for others it comes after a few sessions and this will depend on how much tension a person has in the first place and how quickly they are able to release this tension.

From the outside, there is also a noticeable difference. After Alexander lessons, a person tends to be more upright and can often be physically taller by an inch or more; they have their head more balanced on top of their spine and their shoulders are broader. Their arms tend to move more freely when walking, as do their hip, knee and angle joints. They tend to be naturally more graceful without doing a thing. I can also even hear a big difference as they are walking around the room, as their step is noticeably quieter. The reduction of the jarring of the body that often accompanies every step has a very beneficial effect on the back and neck muscles, as many report that the back pain has noticeably diminished.

People also report a change in their mental, and subsequently their emotional, outlook on life. Within a few lessons, people often tell me that they are calmer, sleeping better and are feeling more at ease with themselves and others. In the next chapter, you will hear from a variety of people who have freed themselves from severe back pain by using the Alexander Technique.

– 14 –

THE POWER OF THE ALEXANDER TECHNIQUE

The Alexander Technique really works. I recommend it enthusiastically to anyone who has neck pains or back pain. I speak from experience.

Roald Dahl

Before we finish I thought it would be useful for you to read some accounts from several other people who have suffered with serious back pain and how they overcame their problem using the Alexander Technique. I thought it would be more beneficial for you to read their accounts in their own words. Some of them are my own pupils, while others were studying the technique 20 years before I had even heard of it, and others I have never met personally.

Giora Pinkas

I met Giora Pinkas in Oxford at an international Alexander teachers' meeting in 2004; he had travelled from his home near San Francisco and had been teaching the technique to others for nearly 40 years. As we got talking he told me of the horrific parachute accident when he was hardly out of school that led him to have Alexander lessons in the first place. This is his story:

I was born in the British Mandate for Palestine before it became Israel. Even in my youth I was very interested in movement of one kind or another and during my school years I excelled in Israeli folk dance and athletics and became among the best at both in Israel. When I left school in 1959 I, like many other men in Israel at the time, went into army for two years' national service. As part of my training I was involved in a freak accident while doing something I would not recommend to anyone: jumping out of an airplane in the pitch dark at night! A squad of parachuters were on a night-time routine military exercise and one by one we all jumped out of the airplane and I was the last to jump. I stepped out of the plane's door, as I had done several times before, but instead of falling towards the ground, I found myself dangling in space, feet up and head down. Somehow my foot had got tied to my rifle, which had flipped and was caught in the door and had halted my fall!

I am not sure how long it took before I realized the seriousness of my predicament, but it felt to me like ages – enough time for my whole young life to be paraded before me – as I contemplated the inevitable: the fact that the pilot would not realize what had happened and would land the plane, which would have been surely the end of me. Luckily, however, there were two highly skilled soldiers on the plane who noticed what happened and, holding onto each other, were able to catch my stretched hand and pull me back into the plane. I was somewhat relieved to say the least, but my relief did not last for long as they immediately made me get ready for another jump!

In the army, as many will know, you do not question orders, you just follow them. That second jump was certainly more successful then the first in one way: I did leave the plane this time, but, probably owing to the previous incident, my parachute's strings were wound too tightly (as in a playground swing) and as a result the canopy got smaller and smaller as I was falling. Although it was very dark and I could not estimate the exact speed and distance, I knew I was falling much faster than normal. It was not long before I hit the ground with a tremendous force. Lying quietly in a field, I knew something was very wrong as I could not feel my legs at all – I even had to touch them gingerly with my hands to see if they were still there!

But to tell the truth, I did not dwell too long on how my body was – I felt very excited and happy just to be alive after such a terrible ordeal and I could not wait to rejoin my friends who had jumped before me and to complete the military exercise that we were all participating in.

However, I soon realized that I had paid a high price for that freak accident as my whole body had suffered an enormous physical shock, which I mainly felt in my feet, ankles and back. In actual fact, I was not the same person after the accident. As time passed I began to notice more and more the non-physical effects of the accident and experienced first-hand that the body and mind are so closely interwoven. I could no longer concentrate my mind and became very restless and unhappy. I returned to dance and music, which partly restored my physical and mental well-being, but my dance training was interrupted by my father's death as I had to go home to look after the family business, and it was not long before my back problem returned. When things had settled down again I took up physical education and dance again to try to recapture my physical and mental wellbeing, but for some reason it did not work a second time and I struggled severely with the pain in my back. Seeing that I was in so much pain, the head of physical education recommended 'a man who had just returned from London' who might be able to help.

This man just happened to be Israeli's very first Alexander Technique teacher Shmuel Nelken who had recently been trained by Patrick Macdonald, one of the very first Alexander teachers.

Within a few lessons I experienced very profound physical, mental and emotional changes were taking place and I soon started to feel very contented; very quickly I had a strong intuition about the huge potential of the technique, not only for back sufferers but for all sorts of mental, emotional and physical problems. In fact I was so impressed with the remarkable effects of the Alexander Technique that I decided to go to London and train with Patrick Macdonald the following year. I have never looked back.

Caroline Martin

I first met Caroline Martin from Galway while I was giving a weekend course at Chrysalis in County Wicklow in Ireland. She followed up the weekend with some individual lessons and then joined the Alexander Teacher Training Course, Galway in 2002. This is her account:

I started to suffer with back pain and sciatica in my mid-twenties. It was extremely painful and was worse at night and it stopped me from sleeping. I had treatment from one osteopath and then another and then tried massage, yoga and reflexology, but nothing seemed to shift the pain for any length of time. I'm not sure if there was a connection, but I was also suffering from really bad menstrual cycles. It was very painful, there was heavy bleeding and the cycle was very irregular. My doctor diagnosed a condition called polycystic ovarian syndrome and said that my womb was inverted; he also told me that my pelvis was out of alignment and there was no chance of having children naturally. After four miscarriages it seemed that he was right.

It was during my late twenties that I first heard of the Alexander Technique and went to a weekend course to learn what it was all about. The theory made perfect sense to me, but it was only when I went to individual sessions that I began to realize what I was doing to myself. When standing I had a habit of leaning backwards and throwing my pelvis forward and digging my heels into the ground. I had always noticed that the heels of my shoes were well worn, but up to now I hadn't realized why. After my first individual lesson I became much more aware of how I was holding my body; I came away feeling lighter and freer and with a greater sense of the spatial awareness. There was a noticeable change in my height as I had to lower my car seat in order to drive home. After a few individual and group sessions, I could feel myself releasing the tension in my lower back, and the sciatica and back pain started to disappear. One of my Alexander teachers, Barbara Conable, showed me that my pelvis was twisted and after some weeks it began to right itself and my periods became less painful, less heavy and the cycle became much more regular. I am happy to say that since that time I have conceived twice naturally and had absolutely no back pain right through the pregnancy. The lasting effects on the technique have given me more energy and have made me a more confident person. I have no hesitation in recommending it to anyone as I honestly feel I owe it to the Alexander Technique that I now have two healthy children.

Rome Godwin

I have never met Rome Godwin from London. She had heard that I was writing a book on the Alexander Technique and back pain and offered me her own case history; this is what she had to say:

I was born in Washington, DC and lived for some years as an adult in Australia and Spain; otherwise I am a Londoner through and through! During my early forties I started to have back problems while working as a manager of a large housing co-operative in London. Over a four-year period I had a bad back, which actually seized up completely three times, and eventually I was getting very bad-tempered with the pain – it was really affecting my life. When in pain I felt as though my whole torso was being drawn in very tightly and often I was unable to stand up from sitting without pain; I was also unable to sit down from standing without terrible pain. Sometimes I was virtually unable to walk, and when I was a passenger in the car in which a friend was conveying me to an osteopath, I yelped each time the car went over a bump. After the last bad attack, I thought: 'I can't continue like this, with my back seizing up every two years' and was determined to find a solution.

In hindsight I know now that my back problem was a direct result of poor posture, but I did not realize this at the time, despite being regularly told by my Mum to 'stand up straight'. She made the mistake of telling me to walk down the street as though it cost £100 to speak to me, and of course I thought that was a dreadful idea and did exactly the opposite! My chest was concave, I had rounded shoulders with a 'sway' back, and an overarched lumbar spine. I personally think that insecurity must have had a lot to do with it, because growing up I had always seemed to be an outsider.

Up until then I had been to an osteopath and been 'sorted out' after a couple of visits, but the trouble was that, although the osteopath was very good, the back pain kept on returning. So finally I rang an actor friend of mine who had been praising the technique very highly and had suggested that I tried it out. So I finally said to him: 'I want that Alexander Technique you've talked about, give me the telephone number!'

When I first saw the very pleasant lady that my friend had recommended I could not understand why it should be called a lesson, because she did not seem to me to be teaching me anything, although the sessions did leave me feeling good. It was a great relief, however, that someone at last was seeking to help me with my on-going back problem. Soon I had other really good Alexander teachers and many lessons followed over the years. These gave me a deeper understanding of what the body is and can do; my upper torso changed shape first, now becoming much straighter – no longer concave with my spine bent and my shoulders pulled in; and then my lower back became flat and strong. The Alexander Technique has made me fitter, calmer and more confident, and I now (usually!) pause for a moment before I act, which lets me be active with almost no tension or confrontation. As well as my body shape dramatically changing, I now have a greater ease of movement and two years ago I started ballet classes at over 60 years of age! . . . Life is good!

Veronica O'Shaughnessy

Veronica O'Shaughnessy from Galway in Ireland was one of my own pupils, who came after many years of severe debilitating backache; within a couple of months of discovering the Alexander Technique her life had dramatically changed for the better. This is her experience:

For more than 15 years I was one of the statistics that suffered from periodic chronic back pain. I would be great for months and then – bang! It would snap or seize in some way, completely compromising my movements. There was no warning or twinge – just gone, couldn't move. It happened at the obvious times like bending or getting out of the shower or in the garden: all the things you would expect as a back sufferer. Then gradually the pain stayed: a niggle became a twinge, the twinge turned into pain, affecting my work and my sleep at night.

This would necessitate a trip to the doctor initially for painkillers; however, due to the side effects of those, I tried alternative methods. My friend recommended a chiropractor in the local town so I travelled to him and, hey presto, I walked out of his building without pain for the first time in a long time.

My trips continued, firstly every six months, and then gradually they became more and more frequent, and the thought of his impulse gun on my lower back brought a sense of dread to my whole body as it was becoming increasingly painful, so I plodded along – suffering not so much in silence, but moaning to the whole world or at least to those who would listen.

The situation worsened and my shoulder locked one day while I was driving and the pain was so intense that it made childbirth feel like a walk in the park. I went to my GP, who gave me anti-inflammatory and pain-relief tablets, and they worked for a week. As soon as I stopped taking them the pain returned in force. I revisited the GP, who decided it was time to call in the big guns and suggested that I see a specialist in one of the Dublin hospitals. 'Great,' I said with delight, 'I am free tomorrow' – only to be told it didn't work like that. He was a busy man and I would have to wait. 'How long?' I asked with dread. Anything between three and five months, was the answer, so having health insurance and being in pain were minor details.

After 13 weeks I was called to see the revered man (who I now thought was God), who was going to cure my back and my shoulder. He took a look at my shoulder, and asked how long I had had it. After explaining about my back and shoulder and going through tests, he informs me that I needed an operation on my back to fix the problem. 'It will be about three months before I can fit you in,' he said. He gave me a list of exercises and said his goodbyes. I was on the list. I took one look at the exercises and thought if I could do those exercises I would have no need for you, Mr Wonderful Doctor.

Man, did I have questions! What if . . .? Will it . . .? But no answers. Right time to see someone else, I thought – get a second opinion.

A week later I met a friend who had had a long suffering backache, but had managed to avoid surgery by using the Alexander Technique and could not believe the improvement. She suggested that I might try it out.

I will give it a try, I thought, nothing to lose. At least he is not going to slice me up and say, 'You may be worse after the operation.'

My first Alexander consultation was one of amazement. My teacher was so confident that all would be well in a few sessions and I almost believed him. I asked him what I had to do to facilitate this miracle and he said very confidently: 'Nothing'. Knowing nothing about the Alexander Technique, my thoughts were 'Right . . . we will see.'

He worked on my shoulders that first visit and for the first in a very long time my shoulder eased and the pain was not as severe.

He explained that the way I was sitting and standing was causing the problem and I was amazed at how much my head weighed. Only then did I realize that 'chin up, chest out' was not the right way to go.

He advised me on sitting in my car and showed me how badly designed my car seat was; he put a wedge-shaped cushion on the seat, which immediately made a huge difference to the pain in my lower back. I now am also the proud owner of a forward sloping chair, which incidentally I love, and sit happily at my desk.

I also bought a pair of VIVOBAREFOOT shoes, which at this stage have clocked up about 50 kilometres. I can feel myself bounce now when I walk instead of just plodding along.

The journey to recovery with the Alexander Technique was a holistic one, and the advice of pausing and thinking before action has changed my life. I found the courage to make some life-changing decisions.

I have changed my career path and am now pursuing something I really love doing. My life has become easier as I am now pain-free most days. I say most days because occasionally I get a twinge and I think, 'Aww, what's happening', and invariably I will find that I missed my semi-supine session for a day or two. The time I spend lying flat with my book under my head has become my oasis of tranquillity. It stills the mind and allows healing in other areas of my life as well. I see things more clearly while allowing my body to be still and lengthened. I have no doubt that it helps in the rejuvenation of your spine by resting it; however, I believe it goes deeper and allows you to connect with what your body needs and is a little quite time in this busy world.

I got called two weeks ago for my operation and I had great pleasure in replying: 'Thank you, however I am happy to inform you I have made a complete recovery without surgery or drugs.'

For me the most important thing of all was that I understood why my lower back ached and why my shoulder was painful. When I changed how I sat, got up from a chair, or bent down to pick something up, everything started to improve.

Thank you seems such an insipid word for the comfort I have received from my treatments – it is a very holistic experience in body, mind and spirit and it is in my life to stay!

Bill Benham

I met Bill Benham, from Salisbury in the UK, recently in La Gomera, one of the Spanish Canary Islands. It was a small gathering of Alexander teachers from all over the world. While having breakfast one morning,

Bill told me how, as a professional musician, he was 'playing through the pain' when he came across the Alexander Technique:

I came from a musical family and from a very early age used to play the piano. When I was nine I took up the violin as well, which has subsequently caused me a great deal of problems since. I was playing in an orchestra from the age of 12, and at 15 was entering the BBC and Carl Flesch competitions. Music has become a huge part of my life. When I was 19 I started to feel first neck and then back pain; it started right between my shoulder blades but quickly spread to the lower back. During a tour in Florida with the London Symphony Orchestra my neck seized up completely and my right wrist became immovable, but like the majority of other musicians I've played through the pain. I was only 22 at the time!

I was very close to giving up the violin altogether and in my desperation I went to see a woman named Jean Gibson who taught an Alexander-Technique-based system of education, which did help my condition. She helped me to start thinking about the height of my chin rest and different kinds of chair, which did help a little. I also used massage and yoga to alleviate some of the pain, but nevertheless I played for the next five years with the London Symphony Orchestra frequently in pain, although it was a little bit more under control. When I was 28 I got a job as co-leader with the Northern Sinfonia Orchestra and in the audition I had to play with a piece of string around my neck to support my violin, which gave me enough relief from the pain to get me the job. My back and neck pain continued, however, and I was advised by one of the horn players in the orchestra to have Alexander lessons with Vivien Mackie, who besides being an Alexander teacher had trained with the famous cellist Pablo Casals.

The release of muscle tension that Vivien was able to impart directly helped me to be completely free of pain for the first time

155

in many years. She showed me how I was over-tensing my muscles every time I played and helped me to stop my habit of trying too hard when playing. She also introduced me to fellow violin player and Alexander teacher Paul Collins, who helped me to see how important it was to change the way I held and supported my violin: by doing so, I could play with much less tension. Believe it or not this was a subject that has never been discussed since I started playing at the age of nine. Through a series of individual and group lessons in the Alexander Technique I have been able to play the violin with very little discomfort or pain in my back and neck. It really has enabled me to carry on my very successful musical career for over 30 years, performing in concerts, festivals and for film and TV.

Sara Shepherd

Although born in Hemel Hempstead in England, Sara Shepherd had spent a long time in Australia before she returned to Europe several years ago: first to France and then to Ireland, where I met her. She was one of a huge number of nurses who are afflicted with back pain on a daily basis as they endeavour to help others. This was her journey to the Alexander Technique:

For most of my adolescence, I knew I would be a nurse. It meant a way of leaving home whilst getting an education, earning money and doing a worthwhile job. It came as a surprise, however, when the doctor in charge of my pre-nursing medical pointed out what he called my 'hyperlordosis', which simply meant I had an exaggerated arch in my lower back, as I had been waitressing throughout my teens and had never experienced back trouble.

On beginning my hospital training, the first nine weeks was given to the basics of basic care. I paid particular attention to the afternoon when we were taught the correct way to lift by the physiotherapist. All the trainee nurses on the course spent the next few days practising our shoulder lifts on each other. However, lifting real patients, who were experiencing pain, fear and anxieties, along with illnesses and disabilitie,s was very different altogether from lifting healthy people or inanimate objects. Within weeks of working on a ward my back would feel tired after every shift. After a year, like almost all the other nurses in training, I had a chronic low-grade backache. Chronic backache can be like background 'noise', you get so used to it that you may not notice it, until it's turned off.

Sometime early in my training, I read my first book on the Alexander Technique. It made sense to me and although I didn't seek out lessons, as there weren't any being taught in my region, I started lying down in the semi-supine position after a heavy shift. The semi-supine helped me to turn off the internal 'noise' of my backache. It also seemed to help me both revive my energy and help me to sleep better.

During the 1980s patient-lifting machines were available, but they were far from plentiful in the hospitals and frankly they were considered time-consuming for nurses and undignified for patients. Before lifting policies were brought into hospitals, we would use them only as a last resort. In my second year of training the slide board was experimented with to slide transfer patients between beds and trolleys. These were safe, easy to use, did not compromise dignity and were cheap. Soon every ward had one and I'm sure the slide board has helped to save many a nurse's and orderly's back.

Along with lifting and transferring patients from chairs to beds, etc., nursing involves a huge amount of bending: from drying between toes and putting on slippers to making beds, giving bedpans, dressing wounds – the endless tasks of a nurse involve continuous bending and are often made much worse by the time pressures due to there being minimal staff. Although the risk of backache was increased by my lumbar hyperlordosis and my tendency to hold tension in my lower back, the worse thing in my opinion, however, was the perpetual bending from the top of the hip rather than at the hip joint itself. Although we studied a great deal of basic anatomy and had been taught manual handling, I still had no idea what it felt like to bend at the hip joint, as we are anatomically designed to. I am convinced that most of the damage to my back came from my poor use in the more incidental repetitive tasks of nursing.

There was one incident that stands out in my mind. It happened at the end of a late shift: I had worked for ten days in a row and was walking a heavy, elderly man back from the toilet when he slipped and lost his footing. I quickly reached out and caught him in an awkward sideways hold and prevented him from falling to the ground. Calling for help and unable to sustain the support of his weight, I began lowering him slowly toward the floor. With the help of a colleague, we coaxed him into a wheelchair and back to bed. This incident was followed by my first real back pain. The low-grade tolerable ache had been replaced by a sharp, searing, twisting pain. It felt like a pinching in my right buttock and radiated down my right leg and throbbed worryingly behind my right knee.

In the 1980s we would admit patients with severe back pain and keep them in traction for weeks, but then when further research came out it showed traction to be no more effective than bed rest. So bed rest is what I chose, with long bouts of semi-supine. After my three days off my back still hurt when I moved so I visited a doctor who told me I had 'slipped a disc'. He told me to keep doing the semi-supine procedure as it seemed to be helping and gave me a week off work to do it. So my back pain healed itself just with rest and after a week I cautiously returned to the wards.

Like many nurses and trainee nurses of my day, I would regularly visit a chiropractor. They were popular in Australia at the time, and during or after a visit I would feel some relief, One afternoon tea break there was a whispered commotion as many nurses crowded around an accident emergency nurse, who had been relaying a detailed account of admitting a young patient unable to walk, control his bladder and barely move his hands following over-exuberant cervical chiropractic manipulation. Although this was a very rare occurrence, my flirtation with chiropractic 'adjustments' ended abruptly then: I did not want to take the chance no matter how small that risk was. I decided that I could live with my backache!

After eight years of nursing I was becoming disillusioned with the reductionistic hospital system, however, and so left for a district nursing position. Although I really loved this work, my back didn't! Working within the confined space of a patient's bathroom proved far trickier and more challenging than the purpose-built rooms at the hospital. I ached from first thing in the morning to the last thing at night and so for the sake of my health I decided to leave nursing. Having always found paperwork to be the most tedious and loathsome part of my work, I knew that, although I had no other qualifications, the thought of office work was repellent. However, I found a job as a sales rep for a pharmaceutical company and before long it became my job to persuade doctors to prescribe more of my company's drugs – that's how averse I was to working in an office!

The hours were brilliant, the money good, they gave me a company car and expenses, but I felt that I had completely sold out. I had willingly sold my soul and would have been fine about it if only my backache had dissipated, even just a bit. All the sitting in waiting rooms and car seats seemed to make it worse than ever, or was it the guilt of leaving nursing? Perhaps this was simply the time to feel it? One day I was reaching into the car boot for my briefcase and just couldn't straighten up. The pain was excruciating. I cancelled my appointments and was seen by one of the doctors in the surgery that I was just about to call on. Again the GP told me I had a 'slipped disc' and referred me to an orthopaedic surgeon. He in turn confirmed their diagnosis and recommended a laminectomy. Laminectomy is an orthopaedic spine operation to remove the portion of the vertebral bone called the lamina. This I knew I didn't want. When district nursing I had called daily on a man who had undergone several such operations and he said that the scar tissue had left him with more severe pain than before his first operation. Surgical outcomes for such conditions are way less predictable than doctors would like and with my medical knowledge I knew it was not worth the gamble.

Instead I booked into a six-week introductory course on the Alexander Technique, favouring the gentler approach. This it turns out was exactly the right thing to do as I found out I was pregnant. The things I learned helped me to manage my back during pregnancy, simple practical things like unlocking my knees, finding my feet and easing off effort. When my son was born, like many little boys, he much preferred to be carried than to be in the pram. I finally sought out individual lessons in the Alexander Technique.

I remember clearly that first gentle yet profoundly deep touch that lightened my head, and eased my back all at once. It seemed like magic. My teacher wasn't very forthcoming with information or telling me how she did it, she simply mumbled something about the quality of the touch being important, but I knew I had found my calling. When my little boy was old enough to go into a nursery school, I began to train as an Alexander Technique teacher. It has been more than a decade since I have experienced back pain, backache belongs to my past and I now get deep satisfaction teaching other people with back pain – particularly showing other nurses to bend into what Alexander called the 'positions of mechanical advantage', so that the deep postural muscles can do their work as nature intended.

Katrina Kenny

Katrina Kenny from Galway, Ireland was another of my own pupils who came to me after having a back problem for over twenty years. Within a few weeks she could feel the pain was receding and referred more people to the Alexander Technique than I can remember. Like myself she really could not believe how simple and effective it was. This is what she had to say:

I have suffered from chronic lower back pain for over 20 years. I am convinced that this was a result of bad posture and my job in a shop, which involved standing for eight hours a day. It came to the stage when I honestly couldn't stand for longer than 10 minutes without feeling the pain in my back. This had a terrible effect on my everyday life, both at home, looking after my children, and at work. After trying one remedy after another, including physiotherapy, back massage and going to my GP, I really thought there was no cure, and tried to come to terms with the fact that I would just have to live with this. I managed by taking pain killers and just accepted that I was destined to a life of pain.

When I started to develop shoulder and neck problems as well I got worried. I was in a lot of pain and the worst thing was the restriction of my movement. I have three young boys and loved to play basketball and bowling with them. When I couldn't play with my children anymore I decided that I needed to go back to the doctor, who sent me for an MRI scan. The result of the scan showed many problems with my shoulder, including chronic impingement syndrome, degenerative joint disease and rotator cuff tendonitis. I was referred to a specialist and he advised surgery. Although I agreed to the operation as a last resort, I was very, very nervous about surgery!

Thankfully for me, it was while I was waiting for my surgery date that I came across a book about the Alexander Technique. After reading the book I had a hope that this could be the answer to my back, neck and shoulder problems.

I went to an Alexander Technique teacher and he said I needed two things for the technique to work: discipline and patience. He told me that that he thought that my lower back would be cured quite quickly, but my shoulder might take a little longer. Even after only a few sessions I was really delighted with the technique, as the first thing I realized I needed to do was not another set of exercises, but to really rest my poor tired body and start to improve my posture. From the first lesson I had such confidence that the technique was going to work for me that I went straight home and cancelled my surgery.

I am delighted to say was that my lower back started to improve very quickly and I have no pain at all now, and my neck and shoulder are also nearly perfect now. It is so wonderful to have a pain-free body again after all those years of being in pain. As an added bonus I also have much more freedom of movement. The thing I really love about the technique is you do not suffer while your body heals itself. It's just a simple matter of correcting bad postural habits, going about everyday tasks with more care, and taking time out of my day to rest my body when it needs it. I am still amazed to think that something so simple could have such a profound effect on my life. I am so glad to have discovered the Alexander Technique and extremely grateful to my Alexander Technique teacher for helping me to relieve my back problems. I can honestly say that my whole life has changed for the better since I started practicing the Alexander Technique. Just recently I went to see a Bruce Springsteen concert in Dublin, which involved standing in a queue for one and a half hours while waiting for tickets and then standing for another three hours at the concert itself, and I can honestly say that I did not have one twinge, ache or pain during the whole time. That is what I call a miracle!

Stephanie McDonald

I also met Stephanie McDonald of Kildare, Ireland on a weekend course that I was running. Again she had a long-standing back problem, and was so impressed with the effectiveness of the technique that she eventually decided to come to Galway to do the training course in order to help others in pain. This is her own account of what happened:

My back pain first began at the age of 19. I was a college student in Dublin at the time. One day I was walking home from college when all of a sudden my back seized up for apparently no reason. Looking back it must have been connected to poor posture, as I remember my mother frequently saying: 'Would you ever stand up straight?' The pain that day was so acute that I could barely get home and when I did my father took me straight away to the casualty department in the local hospital. I had an X-ray taken and when the radiologist read the results he told me I had a slight scoliosis (abnormal lateral curvature of the spine). He then referred me to a physiotherapist and an orthopaedic consultant. The physiotherapist said that I had one leg shorter than the other and gave me an insole to wear in my shoe. The orthopaedic consultant told me that 80 per cent of the population had back pain and wasn't I lucky not to be paralysed. He gave me a cortisone injection into my lower back, which actually made the pain worse.

My pain continued to get worse despite wearing the insole in my shoe. The pain, which was mostly in my lower back, was now affecting me on a day-to-day basis. It had also spread into my shoulders. I also noticed that my pain became worse when I was stressed. After putting up with the pain for two years I decided to try other therapies. I first went to see a spinologist, then an osteopath, followed by many chiropractors. One of the chiropractors told me that one of my legs was not shorter after all and that I had a twisted pelvis. I began to wonder if the twist in my pelvis had been caused by wearing an insole in my shoe for two years! I used to experience relief from my pain for a few days after these visits, however the pain always returned and sometimes with a vengeance. The chiropractor felt that his work was not proving effective because my muscles were too tense and that because of this they were continually pulling the bones of my spine out of place. At this point I had developed neck pain to add to my shoulder and back pain, and it became an effort just to hold my head up as it just felt so heavy. Over time I was getting much worse rather than better.

I then tried a reflexologist and, like the spinal adjustments, I would gain relief, but it would never last more than a week and I began to resign myself to a life of pain. A friend of mine had heard Eamon Dunphy, the famous footballer and sports commentator, speaking on the radio about how the Alexander Technique had helped him with his life-long back problem; my friend thought that it might help me too. I started to have Alexander lessons in Dublin and after each lesson my body felt lighter and freer. After ten lessons most of my pain had melted away. At this point I moved away from Dublin, to a place where there was unfortunately no Alexander teacher. After a few months I noticed that my muscular tension was beginning to creep back in. I realized I had not had enough lessons to be able to help myself.

I decided to go on a residential weekend where the Alexander Technique was taught in a group. It was by watching other people arching their back and pulling their heads back onto their spines during simple actions like standing, walking or getting out of a chair that I saw that I was actually causing my own back pain! I also became aware that the personal stress I had being experiencing in my life was a big contributing factor to the pain I was experiencing in my body. All of this was a huge realization for me. Finally I could see light at the end of the tunnel and felt optimistic that there was a solution to my pain. Up to this point I had been looking for someone to fix me, but now I realized I would have to play an active role in preventing the habits that were causing my back pain. I was so impressed with the power of the technique on that weekend that I decided to train as an Alexander teacher.

I very rarely have back pain these days. The only time I experience any discomfort is usually after I have allowed myself to become stressed, or when I haven't remembered to 'stay present' to myself. On these occasions, I know exactly what I need to do. I return to the principles of the technique and, using my mind, I consciously release the muscular tension. Usually within an hour my back pain has gone.

Studying the Alexander Technique brought me on a profound journey of self discovery, which still continues today. It has changed me not just physically but emotionally and mentally as well. The technique has helped me to be a much more contented person; in fact, I am a very different person to what I was – for the better.

Aino Klippel

I have never met Aino Klippel from Finland, but she heard that I was writing about back pain and offered me her unique story:

Already before school age, I was told my posture wasn't great and I was advised to practice pulling my shoulders back. During my school years my back often hurt when I tried to force my back into the shape of the badly designed school chairs, and my teacher's view of good posture included having a very overarched back. Gradually my back grew into a peculiar shape, but I was constantly reassured that it was 'not a sway back'. I got used to being in some sort of pain all the time and strangely only bending backwards seemed to bring some temporary relief. My shoulders were very tight and I was becoming increasingly short-sighted.

I started playing the clarinet, which was both hard work and rewarding. At home, picking up the clarinet often helped my shoulders to release, and breathing just seemed to take care of itself. I loved the rich sound of my instrument and enjoyed the effortless dance of my fingers on the silver-plated keys. Performing and even orchestra rehearsals or clarinet lessons were compromising my playing quite a lot. When I was anxious to make a good impression, I was trying to both hold my breath and blow at the same time, which caused a lot of tension. I failed to maintain a steady rhythm and struggled with tongue and fingers.

When I began to study music, I moved from the countryside to the city life of Helsinki. Suddenly I had to deal with the constant noise of traffic, pavements and concrete, busy strangers and polluted air. My clarinet sound become narrow, I would quickly run out of breath and my back pain become more intense. Sitting for hours on end through orchestra rehearsals was especially painful. I knew I was doing something wrong with my back but nobody seemed to be able to show me how to go back to normal. My hands started to get cramps, sometimes I had to open the fingers of one hand with the help of the other hand. I got used to waking up with numb arms.

During this time I heard about the Alexander Technique and read a book about it. Because I couldn't find an Alexander teacher, I sought help from experienced clarinettists, massage therapists and a physiotherapist who specialized in musicians. I started to do specific exercises such as stretching, running and swimming. The muscles in my legs and arms were getting stronger, but I had no idea how to use this newly acquired strength for the benefit of my back problem. Trying to follow the physiotherapist's advice and hold myself in a good posture was making my back hurt more than anything else.

I started to look for something else. My massage therapist recommended a yoga class for musicians, which was very gentle and the teacher was truly knowledgeable. I liked his optimistic and educational approach and I started to do yoga every day. It seemed to help me a little in managing pain and stress as well. I enjoyed working in silence, without my instrument.

Over several years I kept working with music and started exploring with increasingly challenging yoga styles. When I saw an advert for an Alexander Technique course for musicians, my only fitness regime at that time was Ashtanga yoga. As a busy, young clarinettist, the yoga had suited me quite well: it was portable, rhythmical, combining breath and movement to gain flexibility and strength. On the other hand the demanding practice was making my muscles even tighter, and now my knees were hurting as well.

The Alexander Technique was something totally different from anything I had tried before. My teacher had very sensitive hands, and she seemed to be able to almost read my thoughts. She explained she could feel when I was tensing my muscles even when I thought I was still just thinking about getting up from a chair. If I could become aware of that reaction, I knew it would lead me towards the more effortless way of being that I remembered so vividly from my childhood. The Alexander lessons were short, but they really helped me to figure things out on my own. Furthermore, the technique didn't require long hours of practice. I could apply it anytime and anywhere.

My Alexander teacher always told me to 'pay some gentle attention to the lower back' Gradually it dawned to me how much I had been compressing that part of my back. Walking on the streets was different: I was looking at the sky as well as the pavement. Some colleagues made compliments about my clarinet sound. My yoga teacher mentioned that there was a pleasant 'juiciness' emerging in my practice.

After a year of Alexander lessons, a cycling accident left me with broken front teeth and a split lower lip. Playing became a real struggle. Problems with my embouchure (the mouthpiece of the clarinet) were challenging the whole of my body, and the fear of having to give up my career was also reflected in my back as it became even more tense. A further two back injuries from unnecessary harsh yoga adjustments also seriously compromised my breathing. I was not in a good state.

I decided to move to London and train at the Alexander Teacher Training School. The first year I hardly played the clarinet and I replaced yoga with long walks across Hyde Park. I loved the training and learned something new every day. I gradually resumed my yoga practice and even though it was exhausting to take regular Ashtanga classes on top of the full-time Alexander training, it really taught me how to look after myself in a demanding environment. Over time both my back and my mind became stronger and back pain became an exception rather than a rule.

Now, two years after graduating as an Alexander teacher I have just returned to my homeland of Finland. Teaching the Alexander Technique is my main occupation, although playing the clarinet feels easier than ever before. When I've been working hard, I have an occasional pain, but it does not go on for days and weeks. I'm also more confident than I used to be – I know that now my back is supporting me rather than me trying to support it.

* * *

These are just a few examples of changes that are possible. The Alexander Technique is not a quick fix and does require you to be actively involved in the process of learning, but the rewards are truly amazing. All you will really need is patience and perseverance. I hope I have conveyed how simple yet profound the Alexander Technique is. It has been a privilege to be able to share some of my experiences with you and I hope that you will try the technique for yourself, especially if, like me, you have had a long-standing back problem, yet have not been able to find the solution to your problem. I sincerely wish you well on your journey to a pain-free life. I would like Alexander to have the last word:

It is essential that the people of civilization should comprehend the value of their inheritance, that outcome of the long process of evolution which will enable them to govern the uses of their own physical mechanisms. By and through consciousness and the application of a reasoning intelligence, man may rise above the powers of all disease and physical disabilities. This triumph is not to be won in sleep, in trance, in submission, in paralysis, or in anaesthesia, but in a clear, open-eyed, reasoning, deliberate consciousness and apprehension of the wonderful potentialities possessed by mankind, the transcendent inheritance of a conscious mind.

RESOURCES

Richard Brennan's websites with useful articles and information about the Alexander Technique:

www.alexander.ie or www.alexandertechniqueireland.com

The Alexander self help tape
This is the perfect accompaniment to *Back in Balance* and gives clear and concise instructions on:

- How to eliminate unwanted tension
- How to prevent or relieve back pain
- How to improve your breathing
- How to practice the two Alexander principles of inhibition and direction
- How to stay in the present moment

This audio cassette costs £15 (US$25 or €19) including postage and packing, and is available from Richard Brennan, Kirkullen Lodge, Tooreeny, Moycullen, Co. Galway, Ireland or by visiting www.alexander.ie/audio.html.

Wedge cushions
For details of good-quality wedge cushions for cars and chairs (not sofas) as described in chapter three, please visit www.alexander.ie/cushion.html.

For supportive chairs that are good for your back please visit:
www.alexander.ie/chairs.html
For well-designed writing desks that slope forward and help to prevent back pain please see Aalborg Desk:
www.aalborgdk.com

Footwear
Details of footwear designed with the Alexander Technique in mind, as mentioned in chapter ten, can be found at www.vivobarefoot.com.

Readers of *Back in Balance* can get 20% off all shoes by using a special promotional code 'Alex20' on this website.

In Ireland please visit www.footwear.ie

Direction *magazine*
Direction Magazine is a wonderful magazine publishing articles and information for teachers and students of the Alexander Technique. Visit the website for free audios, articles, live interviews, plus 25 years of back issues in stock: www.directionjournal.com.

Society of Teachers of the Alexander Technique
The international societies of teachers of the Alexander Technique below give details of how to find a teacher nearest to you. All teachers listed on these websites have undergone extensive three-year training.

For UK please visit:
www.stat.org.uk
For Ireland please visit:
www.isatt.ie
For the rest of the world please visit:
www.alexandertechniqueworldwide.com

INDEX

Index

Index

Index